ELIZABETH IDOWU

I'M PREGNANT...
Now What?

Everything you need to know about pregnancy, birth and beyond

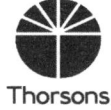

Thorsons

The information provided in this book is for educational and informational purposes only and is not intended as a substitute for professional medical advice, diagnosis, or treatment. Always seek the advice of your doctor or other qualified healthcare provider if you have any questions regarding a medical condition or treatment you know you have or suspect you may have. All efforts have been made to assure the accuracy of the information contained in this book as of the date of publication. However, please note that medical information can change over time, and you should always seek to verify current medical standards.

Never disregard professional medical advice or delay in seeking it because of something you have read in this book. The author and publisher are not responsible for any adverse effects or consequences resulting from the use of any suggestions, preparations or procedures discussed in this book and disclaim all liability in relation to the same. Reliance on any information provided in this book is solely at your own risk. If you think you are having a medical emergency, call the emergency services immediately.

Thorsons

An imprint of HarperCollins*Publishers*

1 London Bridge Street

London SE1 9GF

www.harpercollins.co.uk

HarperCollins*Publishers*

Macken House, 39/40 Mayor Street Upper

Dublin 1, D01 C9W8, Ireland

First published by Thorsons 2026

1 2 3 4 5 6 7 8 9 10

© Elizabeth Idowu (Mamadinya) 2026

Elizabeth Idowu asserts the moral right to be identified as the author of this work.

A catalogue record of this book is available from the British Library.

ISBN 978-0-00-873515-9

Printed and bound in the UK using 100 per cent renewable electricity at CPI Group (UK) Ltd.

All rights reserved. No part of this publication may be reproduced, stored in a retrieval system, or transmitted, in any form or by any means, electronic, mechanical, photocopying, recording or otherwise, without the prior written permission of the publishers.

Without limiting the exclusive rights of any author, contributor or the publisher of this publication, any unauthorised use of this publication to train generative artificial intelligence (AI) technologies is expressly prohibited. HarperCollins also exercise their rights under Article 4(3) of the Digital Single Market Directive 2019/790 and expressly reserve this publication from the text and data mining exception.

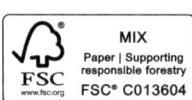

For every mother and baby still to come. May your journeys be safer, softer and supported at every step.

CONTENTS

Introduction	*1*
PART 1: The First Trimester	5
PART 2: The Second Trimester	91
PART 3: The Third Trimester	131
PART 4: The Big Push (Literally)	167
PART 5: Postpartum	261
Endnotes	*299*
Glossary	*303*
Resources	*307*
Acknowledgements	*309*
About the Author	*313*

INTRODUCTION

Let me start by saying – I'm a reader. A proper one. I love books; I love words; I love the way they can transport you or ground you. And even though I live online, chatting away on Instagram and TikTok, I've always been big on going to the *right* place for the *right* information. That's what this book is. A lot of thought, care and a *ridiculous* amount of research have gone into every page.

But before we dive into the first trimester, I want to pause here. I want to pause with *you*. Because I can't even begin to imagine all the different journeys that might have led you to this page. Maybe this is your very first positive pregnancy test. Maybe this is your rainbow baby. Maybe you've been through IVF (In Vitro Fertilisation) and you finally have your baby growing inside you. Maybe you just tried once and bam – you're pregnant. Or maybe the pull-out method stopped working for you. Or maybe you're not even pregnant yet – just planning ahead for when you are . . . or you're just nosy, and honestly, that's fine too. I could go on forever, but you get my gist.

And no matter how you got this book, however it ended up in your hands, what's important is that it's here, with you. Maybe you went out and bought it because you wanted to invest in yourself. Maybe it was a thoughtful gift from your best friend. Maybe your partner handed it to you, hoping it would help answer the million questions bouncing around. Or maybe a family member slipped it into your lap as a not-so-subtle hint that it's time to get stepping (don't worry, we'll talk about boundaries later in the book).

Whatever the route, you're here now – so let's get into it.

When it comes to pregnancy, it's not just about facts; it's about feelings. And I want you to feel held, seen, reassured and maybe even a little entertained while you're here. This isn't a book that's going to wipe away every bit of anxiety; I'd never make that kind of promise. But I do hope that every now and then, you'll read a sentence and go: 'Oh my goodness – yes! That's *exactly* what I'm feeling.' Or maybe even: 'Oh wow, I'm so glad I didn't go through that.'

Whether it's laughter, clarity or a sense of being less alone, I hope this book gives you what you need in the moment you need it. I hope it feels like a warm hug when nothing else does. Because pregnancy is massive – not just physically, but emotionally, mentally and spiritually. And the fact that you've trusted me to be part of your journey? I don't take that lightly.

This isn't a textbook. I'm not here to turn you into midwives. But I *am* here to make sure you walk into this

INTRODUCTION

experience knowing more than you would have if you'd just stuck to googling at 3 a.m. I want you to have *words*. Real words. Medical words. Funny words. And yes – Pringle hand. (You'll find out what that means later, and no – it's *not* what you think.) I want you to feel justified. Educated. Empowered. I want you to feel like you know what's happening, what *could* happen, and that you've got someone in your corner either way.

This book is your safe space. Your secret weapon. Your non-judgemental pregnancy bestie. But it's more than just an info dump; it's a journey, one we're going on together, trimester by trimester. From that first 'Am I . . .?' moment to the first scan, the second trimester stretch, the third trimester waddle, the birth itself – whether that baby's coming out of your vagina or through your stomach (well, technically, your abdomen), I'm with you through it all.

We're going to talk about things no one prepares you for. Like your first pee after birth (yes, that *is* a thing), or the odd symptoms that make you wonder if you're the only one experiencing them. Spoiler: you're not.

But beyond the practical stuff, you'll get to know *me* in these pages. I'm not hiding behind a white coat. I'm a qualified midwife, yes – but I'm also a storyteller, a ranter, a listener and a woman who's had the privilege of working with *thousands* of pregnant women. I'm not a mum yet myself, but I've been in the room when lives have changed. I've held hands, wiped tears, cheered women on as they birthed their babies – and I've learned *so* much from them. You'll hear their stories throughout this book. You'll meet some of the women I've supported in pregnancy. You'll laugh with them, relate to them and maybe even cry with them. And I hope I do their stories justice.

Everything in here - the knowledge, the tips, the side notes, the humour, the honesty - it all comes from years of listening, supporting, learning and showing up. And I've made sure it's presented in a way you can actually digest. Because pregnancy is already overwhelming enough, this book shouldn't be.

So, thank you. Thank you for letting me be part of your pregnancy. Now, settle in. Laugh when it's funny, cry when it's real and underline the bits you want to come back to.

You've got this - and I've got you.

(That's the cheesiest I'll be in the whole book, I promise!)

PART 1

THE FIRST TRIMESTER

YOU'RE PREGNANT . . . NOW WHAT?

I can't count how many pregnancy reveal videos I've seen on Instagram where women look absolutely stunned that they're pregnant, even though, let's be real, they've been doing the do.

Finding out you're pregnant – whether it's something you actively planned or something that completely blindsided you – can hit with the force of a tidal wave. Excitement, fear, joy, anxiety, disbelief, overwhelm – sometimes all in the span of five minutes. Pregnancy is a huge shift, and no matter how much you prepared for it (*or didn't*), adjusting to the reality of it takes time. However you're feeling right now, it's all valid.

Even if you've been actively trying for a baby – tracking ovulation, taking vitamins and doing everything by the book – that positive test can still feel like a freight train hitting you at full speed. Suddenly, it's real. And then the what-ifs start creeping in. *Am I really ready? Will I be a good parent? What if something goes wrong?*

Even when pregnancy is wanted and planned, that doesn't mean you won't have moments of panic, doubt or feeling totally unprepared. This is a major transition, and feeling both excited and overwhelmed at the same time is completely normal. If you're feeling anxious, take things one step at a time. You don't need to have everything figured out today. Give yourself the space to process it at your own pace, and know that if excitement doesn't hit immediately, that's okay. Some women gradually warm up to pregnancy as things start to feel more real, while others never get that 'glowing-overjoyed' moment – and that's okay, too. Every pregnancy is different.

For some, pregnancy is a complete shock. Maybe you weren't trying, maybe the timing is all wrong or maybe you were convinced you'd be one of those rare exceptions to the 'one time is all it takes' rule. Whatever the case, if you're struggling to process it, that's okay. You might feel scared, unsure or even be mourning the version of your life you thought you'd be living right now. Some people feel guilty for not immediately being happy, but pregnancy isn't just about a baby; it's about your life changing in a way you might not have expected. Give yourself permission to feel *everything*. It's okay if you don't have clarity yet.

Talk to someone you trust, whether it's your partner, a close friend or even a midwife who can offer support and guidance. Many women who were initially unsure about their pregnancy find that their feelings evolve over time, while others may need a longer adjustment period – and that's perfectly fine. Some women even delay their pregnancy bookings (see below) because they need time to decide whether to continue with the pregnancy. There is no one-size-fits-all reaction to finding out you're expecting.

Pregnancy brings big changes – whether planned, unplanned, exciting, terrifying or something in between. You don't need to have all the answers today. Feel what you feel, give yourself grace and trust that however your journey unfolds, you will figure it out in your own time. Whether it's your own expectations or the opinions of others, remember: this is your pregnancy, your journey and no one else gets to dictate how you feel about it.

HEALTH AND MEDICAL

THE BOOKING APPOINTMENT

There are many different tests, appointments and scans you'll be offered throughout your pregnancy. If there are any complications, the frequency of these tests should increase – *should* being the key word here. With the NHS under pressure, this doesn't always happen as smoothly as we'd like, but let's talk about the tests you'll be offered and what we're looking for. If you're going to spend half your pregnancy waiting in hospital corridors, you should at least know what you're waiting for!

I'M PREGNANT ... NOW WHAT?

The first appointment you'll have as a preggo is your booking appointment – the one where we literally add you to the system. It's also the longest appointment you'll have, because we're about to ask you *every question under the sun*. From whether you've ever had chickenpox to whether you and your partner are related by blood (yes, it sounds weird, but we really do ask that!), this appointment covers it all. Some of the questions might seem random – or even pointless – and honestly, some of them are. But you'd be surprised how the most seemingly irrelevant information can help us make a life-saving decision later down the line. So, bear with us – we promise there's a reason for every question! During this appointment, we'll take lots of blood tests. These aren't just for fun; we're checking things like your blood type, Rhesus status, iron levels and whether you're a carrier of sickle cell or thalassaemia. These tests are super important because they give us a baseline to compare future results against, helping us track any changes in your health throughout your pregnancy.

We'll also check your height, weight, blood pressure and CO_2 (carbon dioxide) levels. This helps us identify early risks, like high blood pressure, which could lead to conditions such as pre-eclampsia later. We'll also ask about your mental health and home life. This might feel intrusive, but it's really important. If you've ever struggled with depression, anxiety or any other mental health condition, we need to know so we can support you properly. We'll also ask about

THE FIRST TRIMESTER

your safety at home – and yes, even if your partner is in the room, we'll always find a way to ask when you're alone. If you ever feel unsafe, this is a chance for us to help. Next, we'll talk about your previous pregnancy history (if you've been pregnant before). Did you have complications? Was your baby born early? What did your baby weigh? What country did you give birth in? How much did you bleed last time? Did you tear? Any previous caesarean births? This information helps us plan the right care for you this time around.

Then, there's the infectious disease screening. We'll test your blood for HIV, hepatitis B, syphilis and immunity to rubella (German measles). These are routine tests, and if anything comes up, early treatment can help prevent passing infections to your baby. If your blood type is Rhesus negative (meaning your blood doesn't have a certain protein that most people's blood does), we'll explain why you might need Anti-D injections later in pregnancy to protect your baby if they're Rhesus positive.

We'll also calculate your due date based on the first day of your last period. Don't get too attached to it, though – this date may shift slightly after your dating scan, which happens between 10–14 weeks. We'll talk you through the screening tests you'll be offered, including checks for Down's syndrome, Edwards' syndrome and Patau's syndrome. These are completely optional, and we'll give you all the information you need to decide whether you want them.

I'M PREGNANT ... NOW WHAT?

Finally, we'll ask about your lifestyle – things like smoking, alcohol and drug use (recreational or prescribed). I'd love to say no judgement from us here, but that's not strictly true. We midwives are a nosy bunch. We ask a lot of questions, we observe, we connect the dots. It might look and feel like we're judging you, and, in a way, we are – but everything you tell us informs us on how to look after you, and that's why I'm making sure you know the importance of telling the truth. Let me be clear: our opinions are our opinions, but any good midwife knows that personal beliefs should never interfere with professional care. No matter what choices you make, you deserve to be treated with respect, dignity and the highest standard of support. It's your body, your baby, your choice – we're only here to provide the best care.

Once all that's done, we'll book you in for your next midwife appointments and your 12-week scan. You'll also be given access to your maternity notes, either in a big folder (your pregnancy 'bible') or digitally through the NHS app, depending on your hospital. This is where all your test results, appointment details and pregnancy progress will be recorded – don't lose it!

So, there you have it – the first official step into the world of prenatal care. One long appointment, a million questions and a tiny vial of your blood that tells us everything we need to know about you. But at least now, if you're stuck in the waiting room, you'll know exactly what you're waiting for!

THE FIRST TRIMESTER

FIRST TRIMESTER PHYSICAL CHANGES

For many women, the first trimester comes with all the symptoms but no bump to prove it. It's wild how much is happening inside your body while on the outside everything looks the same. Most women say this is the most symptomatic trimester, and to make things harder, many keep their pregnancy a secret at this stage. That means keeping their struggles a secret too: functioning at work like normal, pretending that someone's overpowering perfume isn't making them gag or acting like they're not running on fumes from sheer exhaustion.

Let's talk about the physical changes you might go through. But before we dive into the nitty-gritty, let's get one thing straight: the mind is powerful. It's easy to read a long list of symptoms and suddenly convince yourself that you're experiencing all of them. That's not how this works. You may not experience every symptom. In fact, you might breeze through the first trimester wondering what all the fuss is about. And if you do experience some of these changes, my goal is to reassure you that there's a reason behind the madness. You're not broken. You're not doing pregnancy 'wrong'. Your body is just working around the clock to grow a life, and that's no small job.

SURVIVING FIRST TRIMESTER EXHAUSTION (WITHOUT DRIBBLING ON YOUR DESK)

If you've spent even five minutes in the pregnancy section of social media, you've probably seen countless posts of women in their first trimester talking about how all they do is sleep. It's the kind of exhaustion that makes you question how you're supposed to function as a human being. One of my friends, a teacher, told me she was in complete denial about being exhausted. *I'm fine,* she thought, until one day, she rested her head on her desk for just a moment. Not to sleep, just to rest. One hour later, she was woken up by a student saying, *Miss, are you okay?* with a pool of dribble on the table. That's how real the exhaustion is. So why can pregnancy make you feel like you've been hit by a truck (aside from the *small* matter of growing a human from scratch)?

- **Hormonal Chaos.** Your progesterone levels skyrocket, making you extra sleepy. It's like your body is drugging you into hibernation mode to make sure you don't overdo it.
- **Increased Blood Production.** Your body is suddenly making up to 50 per cent more blood to support the baby, which can lower your blood pressure and reduce oxygen circulation. Less oxygen = more exhaustion.
- **Blood Sugar and Blood Pressure Drops.** Your body is adjusting, and dips in both can leave you feeling lightheaded, sluggish and just . . . done.
- **Increased Metabolic Rate.** Your body is working overtime to create a whole placenta, which, let's be honest, is pretty impressive. But it also zaps your energy.

THE FIRST TRIMESTER

- **Emotional and Physical Adjustments.** The mix of excitement, stress and anxiety is mentally draining. Add that to the physical changes, and it's no wonder you're wiped out.
- **Disrupted Sleep.** Between frequent bathroom trips, nausea and hormonal chaos, getting a full night's rest feels like wishful thinking.

Basically, your body is doing the absolute most, and you are 100 per cent allowed to feel tired. Now, while you absolutely deserve to rest, most of you are still working and have things to do. So, how do you manage the exhaustion without completely shutting down?

1. **Rest Whenever You Can**
   - Take short power naps if possible. A quick 15–20 minute nap can do wonders.
   - Aim for 7–9 hours of sleep at night.
   - Keep a consistent bedtime routine (*easier said than done, I know, especially if you already have kids – if that's the case, I've got nothing for you*).
2. **Stay Hydrated**
   - Drink water – yes, I know it means more trips to the bathroom, but dehydration makes fatigue worse.
   - Cut back on excess caffeine (no more than 200mg per day, see page 40) – it might feel like your lifeline, but too much can mess with your energy levels in the long run.

3. Fuel Your Body Right
   - Focus on foods that keep you going:
   - Iron-rich foods (spinach, lean meat, beans) to prevent anaemia and combat fatigue.
   - Protein and healthy fats (nuts, eggs, yoghurt) for sustained energy.
   - Complex carbs (whole grains, oats, sweet potatoes) for slow-release fuel instead of sugar crashes.
4. Gentle Movement
   - Short walks, yoga or stretching can help boost circulation and fight fatigue.
   - Fresh air and movement = instant energy boost.
5. Manage Stress and Listen to Your Body
   - Deep breathing, meditation or a pregnancy-safe massage can work wonders.
   - Cut down on commitments and don't push yourself too hard.
   - If you need to say *no* to things, do it – your body is already supporting your baby's development, and that's a full-time job.

BLOATING AND CONSTIPATION: THE UNINVITED GUESTS

If you've ever looked down at your stomach in the first trimester and thought, *Wait, am I showing already?*, there's a good chance it's not a baby bump, it's bloating. Pregnancy

THE FIRST TRIMESTER

bloating is on a different level. And then there's constipation – bloating's toxic boyfriend. If you don't get ahead of it early, it can make you feel even more sluggish and uncomfortable. So, what's causing all of this – and more importantly, what can you do about it?

Let's talk about one of the biggest culprits: progesterone. This hormone is an absolute MVP when it comes to maintaining pregnancy, but it also plays a major role in a long list of symptoms (so you'll hear me mention it a lot). One of its most noticeable effects? Slowing down digestion. Progesterone relaxes the muscles in the digestive tract. This means food moves sluggishly through your intestines. The result? Bloating and constipation. Your digestion is already working more slowly on purpose as the body extracts more nutrients from food during pregnancy to maximise nourishment for the baby. But while this sounds great in theory, it can also cause gas to build up (*hello, bloating*).

As early as the first trimester, the uterus starts expanding and shifting, putting pressure on the intestines. This added pressure makes bowel movements harder to pass, increasing the likelihood of constipation. Then there's iron, another key player. Many prenatal vitamins contain iron because it's essential for red blood cell production, but iron can make stools harder for some people, contributing to constipation. On top of this, because blood volume and fluid needs increase during pregnancy, it's easy to become dehydrated – which can worsen constipation. And if you're not getting enough fibre, digestion slows down even further.

HORMONE CHEAT SHEET

- **hCG (human chorionic gonadotropin):** The 'pregnancy test hormone'. It's made by the placenta in early pregnancy and is what those sticks are picking up when they turn positive. It helps keep the pregnancy going in the very early weeks.
- **Progesterone:** Think of this as the 'protector'. It relaxes your womb muscles so your baby can grow in peace, helps keep the pregnancy stable and also has a hand in preparing your body for labour later on.
- **Oestrogen:** The 'builder'. It helps your womb and placenta grow, boosts blood flow and plays a part in developing the milk ducts in your breasts.
- **Relaxin:** The 'loosener'. It softens your ligaments and joints so your pelvis can open up when the time comes. (It also explains why you might feel a bit wobbly or achy sometimes.)
- **Oxytocin:** The 'love and labour hormone'. It kicks off contractions, helps with bonding and even flows when you cuddle or breastfeed.
- **Prolactin:** The 'milk maker'. It gets your breasts ready to produce milk and keeps the supply going after birth.

THE FIRST TRIMESTER

- **Endorphins:** Your body's natural pain relievers. These rise during labour and help you cope (and they're why people sometimes describe feeling a little euphoric after birth).

BLOATING AND CONSTIPATION HACKS

If bloating and constipation have you struggling, try not to stress. There are simple ways to get things moving again (*yes, pun intended*).

Fibre

Fibre is your best friend. Think of it as the broom that sweeps your digestive system clean. Aim for 25–30 grams a day by loading up on whole grains, prunes, pears, leafy greens and gut-friendly legumes. Now, let me be honest: nothing would tempt me to eat some of the things I'm suggesting. But then again, I'm not pregnant, so maybe that would humble me.

Hydration

Fibre alone won't help if you're not drinking enough water. Try to drink about 8–10 glasses a day to keep digestion flowing smoothly. A warm glass of water first thing in the morning can act like a natural laxative.

Movement
No, you don't need to become an athlete overnight, but a 20–30 minute walk or some gentle prenatal yoga/stretches can wake up a sluggish digestive system.

Natural Supplements
Now, let's sprinkle in some magnesium and probiotics. Foods like avocados, nuts and spinach help keep stools soft and manageable, while probiotic-rich foods like yoghurt and kefir support a healthy gut. If iron supplements are behind your constipation struggles (see page 30), talk to your healthcare provider about switching to a slow-release version – because no one should have to choose between a healthy pregnancy and comfortable digestion.

Simple Diet Adjustments
Finally, if bloating is your biggest issue, cut back on gas-producing foods like carbonated drinks, fried foods and cruciferous veggies (*yes, that means easing up on the broccoli and cabbage*). Smaller, more frequent meals are your friend. Large meals? They'll only add to that bloated, uncomfortable feeling. With a few tweaks (and plenty of hydration), you'll hopefully be back to feeling like yourself in no time – minus the unwanted food baby.

THE FIRST TRIMESTER

PREGNANCY BOOBS: SORE, SWOLLEN AND SERIOUSLY SENSITIVE

A lot of first trimester symptoms feel eerily similar to PMS (Pre-Menstrual Syndrome), which is why so many women feel like their period is about to start, only to realise they're actually pregnant. One of the biggest PMS copycats? Breast tenderness. And for some women, it's so intense that even someone looking at their boobs feels painful. So, who's to blame? Our bestie progesterone and her sister oestrogen. These two are working overtime from the moment you conceive, getting your body ready for breastfeeding – which is hilarious because, at this point, you probably don't even have a bump! But we love a prepared queen, and your breasts are ahead of the game.

From the moment you conceive, oestrogen and progesterone levels soar to support the pregnancy. These hormones kickstart major breast changes, making them feel swollen, sore and extra sensitive. More blood flows to the area, making the tissue tingly and tender. Meanwhile, progesterone encourages the body to retain more fluid, which explains why your boobs suddenly feel fuller, heavier and uncomfortable. The milk ducts start expanding early, prepping for their big debut. This expansion puts extra pressure on the surrounding tissue, making soreness worse. As your breasts stretch and grow, the nerve endings become extra sensitive, which is why simple things like putting on a bra or lying on your side feel unbearable. The *kind-of* good news? Breast tenderness is usually at its worst in the first trimester and often eases by the second trimester as your body adjusts. So, hang in there. Your boobs are just ahead of schedule.

> ### **BREAST PAIN RELIEF**
>
> Let's talk about some hacks to help with tender breasts, because if they're going to be this sore, the least we can do is make them *somewhat* comfortable.
>
> - Ditch the underwire and swap it for a soft, supportive bra. I know this isn't always ideal for my mummies who are *blessed* in the chest, but if the wire is making things worse, let your breasts be free. Maternity and sports bras offer gentle support without digging in, making them a game-changer during the first trimester. Some women say that even turning over in bed hurts, and honestly? I believe them. If that's you, try wearing a lightweight sleep bra – it helps keep things in place and minimises soreness from sudden movements.
> - Stay hydrated and ease up on the salt. Fluid retention can also make breast tenderness worse. Drinking plenty of water and cutting back on processed or extra-salty foods can reduce bloating, not just in your boobs, but *everywhere* else, too.

- Opt for soft, breathable fabrics that don't add unnecessary pressure – your boobs are already under *enough* stress. Tight tops and bras that press against your chest? Absolutely not.
- Lightly massage your breasts with pregnancy-safe oils like coconut or almond oil to improve circulation and ease tightness. Keeping your skin moisturised as your breasts stretch and grow can also help with the discomfort.
- Try a cool or warm compress. You can buy ones that work both ways – stick them in the freezer for a cooling effect or pop them in the microwave for warmth. Try both and see what gives you the most relief.

If the pain is just too much, paracetamol is usually considered safe during pregnancy, but as always, check with your midwife or doctor before taking anything. Remember that breast tenderness usually calms down by the second trimester – so until then, be kind to yourself and honestly, take your bra off the moment you get home.

PREGNANCY AND PEEING: WHY YOUR BLADDER IS WORKING OVERTIME

If you feel like you're living in the bathroom, constantly running back and forth, congratulations – you've unlocked one of the most common early pregnancy symptoms: non-stop peeing. The worst part? A lot of these pees are just the tiniest trickle. Increased urination in the first trimester is completely normal and while it might feel like an inconvenience, your body has a good reason for it.

Hormones, as always, are to blame. But this time we'll cut progesterone some slack. The main culprit here is the pregnancy hormone hCG. It's working overtime, not just to keep your pregnancy going but also to increase blood flow to your pelvic area. This extra circulation stimulates your kidneys, making them work more efficiently to filter waste. More fluid getting processed means more bathroom trips for you. At the same time, your blood volume is surging. Your body is now producing up to 50 per cent more blood to support your growing baby,[1] and with all that extra blood comes extra fluid that needs to be processed. More fluid moving through your kidneys means more fluid leaving your body, so naturally, your bladder works overtime.

Then there's your uterus, which is still small but already making its presence felt. As it expands to make room for the baby, it starts pressing against your bladder. Just a little pressure can make your bladder feel full, even when it's really not. To top it all off, pregnancy increases your thirst, so you're probably drinking more water than usual, which only adds to the cycle. The more I write this book - and mind you, we're only in the first trimester - the more I'm

THE FIRST TRIMESTER

reminded of the power of being a woman. It's easy to look at pregnancy and think, *wow, this is a lot.* But no - look at how your body is working overtime. You are the epitome of strength. Keep that in mind.

It's easy to think, *Maybe I should drink less so I pee less.* Don't even think about cutting back on fluids. Staying hydrated is crucial, not just for your health but for your baby's development. Dehydration can make other pregnancy symptoms, like nausea and headaches, even worse. If night-time bathroom trips are driving you crazy, try drinking more water earlier in the day and easing up right before bed. When you do go to relieve yourself, try leaning forward slightly. This can help empty your bladder more completely so you don't find yourself back on the toilet five minutes later.

The only real concern with all this peeing is the risk of urinary tract infections (UTIs), which are more common during pregnancy. If you notice a burning sensation when you go, cloudy or foul-smelling urine or a constant feeling of needing to pee but barely anything comes out, check in with your healthcare provider.

The good news? This relentless bathroom cycle won't last forever. By the time you hit the second trimester, your uterus will move up and away from your bladder, giving you a bit of relief. Howeverrrrrrrrr ... When you hit the third trimester, it's no longer your uterus causing the problem - it's your baby deciding to use your bladder as a personal trampoline. So, enjoy the break while it lasts.

I'M PREGNANT ... NOW WHAT?

CRAMPING AND SPOTTING

Most of the symptoms I've mentioned earlier are just irritating for most women. But cramping and spotting in early pregnancy? Those symptoms quickly shift the feeling from annoyance to fear, especially for women who have previously experienced a miscarriage or stillbirth. That stomach-tightening panic? We can't pretend it isn't real. Pregnancy isn't always all roses, and the reality is, many women struggle with different aspects of it. The good news is that in most cases, cramping and spotting are completely normal. Your body is undergoing massive changes, and sometimes that comes with a few uncomfortable symptoms. So how do you know when to brush them off and when to call your doctor? Let's break it down.

Your uterus is stretching and growing, making room for the tiny human developing inside. This can cause mild to moderate cramping, similar to period pains. It's usually nothing to worry about and can come and go throughout the first trimester. The increase in progesterone (as we saw on page 16) also relaxes your muscles, which can lead to mild uterine contractions. Constipation can also be a culprit, and trapped gas and slow digestion can cause cramp-like discomfort – and let me tell you, the pain of trapped gas can be intense – making it hard to tell what kind of cramping you're actually feeling.

Some women also experience round ligament pain, a sharp, pulling sensation on one or both sides of the lower

THE FIRST TRIMESTER

belly. This usually happens when you move suddenly, sneeze or stand up too quickly. It's caused by the ligaments supporting your uterus stretching as it grows. Spotting, which is light bleeding that doesn't fill a pad, is fairly common in the first trimester. One of the most common causes is implantation bleeding, which happens when the fertilised egg attaches to the uterine lining – usually around weeks 4–6. Not every woman experiences implantation bleeding, but if you do, it's typically harmless.

Some women also notice spotting after sex or a vaginal exam because pregnancy hormones make the cervix more sensitive and prone to light bleeding. Hormonal shifts can also cause occasional spotting as your body adjusts to pregnancy. If the spotting is light, pink or brownish in colour and isn't accompanied by severe cramps, it's usually nothing to worry about.

If cramping is mild, rest is your best friend. Put your feet up, stay hydrated and try a warm (not hot) compress on your lower belly. Gentle movement, like stretching or prenatal yoga, can help ease discomfort. If constipation is part of the problem, increase your fibre and water intake to keep digestion moving. For spotting, take it easy and avoid strenuous exercise until the bleeding stops. If spotting happens after sex, it's likely nothing to worry about, but you might want to take a break for a few days to see if it resolves.

While mild cramping and light spotting are normal, certain symptoms could signal something more serious.

Call your healthcare provider if:

- Cramping is severe and persistent, especially if it feels like sharp, stabbing pain.
- Bleeding becomes heavy, bright red or fills a pad in an hour.
- You pass large clots or tissue.
- You feel dizzy, faint or experience intense lower back pain.
- The cramping is focused on one side, which could indicate an ectopic pregnancy (a pregnancy outside the uterus, which requires immediate medical attention).

The first trimester is full of weird, unexpected symptoms, and cramping and spotting can be unsettling. But in most cases, they're just part of your body's way of adjusting to pregnancy.

That said, trust your instincts. If something feels off, contact your healthcare provider. Your peace of mind is worth it.

EXCESS SALIVA (PTYALISM)

Now, I was going to leave this one out. Honestly, it's not the most common symptom, and you might never experience it. But I've included it for *one* very important reason: I have trauma.

Let me set the scene.

I was in secondary school, and my auntie Yinka, who was heavily pregnant at the time, came to pick me up in her car.

THE FIRST TRIMESTER

I got in, chatting away, and I spotted a water bottle on the floor of the car. I was thirsty, so naturally, I did what any normal person would do – I picked it up to take a sip.

She *screamed*. Like, full-body, horror-movie-level scream. Why? Because that wasn't water. It wasn't Lucozade. It wasn't even squash.

It. Was. Her. Saliva.

Yes. You read that right. The bottle was full of her spit, because her pregnancy symptom was so bad she physically *could not swallow her own saliva*. And I nearly drank it. So now you understand why I *had* to include this symptom.

The medical name for it is **ptyalism**, and while it's rare, it can be an absolute nightmare. It usually pops up in the first trimester (sometimes linked to nausea), and it's exactly what it sounds like: your body just starts producing a ridiculous amount of spit. Some people have to carry tissues or bottles around. Some literally have to spit every few minutes. It can be that intense.

We don't fully know why it happens – blame hormones, blame the universe – but if it happens to you, just know:

- you're not alone;
- it's *temporary*; and
- you now have my permission to make everyone in your life feel awkward about it.

Chewing gum, sucking ice or nibbling dry crackers can sometimes help. But mostly? It's one of those 'just get through it' symptoms. And hey, at least you're not accidentally drinking someone else's.

PREGNANCY DOS AND DON'TS

BUILDING A BABY FROM SCRATCH: THE NUTRIENTS THAT MATTER AND FOOD SAFETY

There are hundreds of prenatal vitamins out there, each promising your baby will be a genius or the next world leader - but let's cut through the noise and focus on what's actually essential in the first trimester. The first trimester is no joke. Your body is literally hard at work nurturing new life, and the right nutrition makes all the difference. But between morning sickness, food aversions and craving plain bread and crisps like they're a food group, eating a perfectly balanced diet is easier said than done. That's where prenatal vitamins come in - they help fill the gaps when your appetite is playing games with you. But which ones actually matter, and which ones are just extra? Let's talk.

What You Actually Need

Folic Acid (or Methylfolate) - If there's one vitamin you absolutely need, it's this one. Folic acid (one of the eight B vitamins) reduces the risk of neural tube defects like spina bifida, which affect the baby's brain and spine. The recommended dose is 400mcg daily, starting before conception (if possible) and continuing until at least 12 weeks.

THE FIRST TRIMESTER

Now, here's the thing – for years, folic acid was the gold standard. But newer research suggests that over half of women may have a genetic variation called methylenetetrahydrofolate reductase (MTHFR), which makes it harder for their body to properly process synthetic folic acid.[2] The good news is that these women can still process folate – the active form. So if you've been told this applies to you, look for methylfolate, which is easier for your body to absorb and use.

There's nothing to stress about here. A lot of fertility treatments and prenatal vitamins already use folate instead of folic acid, and everyone can absorb folate. So the easiest thing to do is look for a supplement that contains folate – that way you're covered either way.[3]

What's wild is that folic acid started as an anaemia treatment in the 1930s but became a game-changer in prenatal care. Thanks to Lucy Wills (the scientist who discovered it), millions of babies have been born healthier because of this one simple nutrient. The recommended dose of 400mcg is based on limited human trials, mostly because it's ethically tricky to experiment on pregnant women. We do know that 400mcg reduces the risk of neural tube defects by up to 70 per cent – [4] but testing lower doses just to see if they'd still work would be unethical. So, this is one of those cases where, if it isn't broken, don't fix it.

Vitamin D – Let's be honest, in the UK, we barely see the sun. Vitamin D is crucial for bone development and immune function. The NHS recommends 10mcg (400 IU) daily throughout pregnancy.

Iron – Your blood volume increases by 50 per cent during pregnancy, which means iron is working overtime to help carry oxygen to both you and your baby. If your iron levels are low (which is common), you might feel extra tired, dizzy or breathless. Most prenatal vitamins contain 17-27mg of iron, but if you're diagnosed with anaemia, your midwife may recommend a higher dose. A gentle reminder – iron supplements can cause constipation. To help absorption (*and keep your digestion moving*), pair it with vitamin C (think orange juice, strawberries or a squeeze of lemon in your water). Iron tablets also make your poo black, which can be so scary to see the first time – so, no, you're not bleeding internally; it's the tablets.

Iodine – This essential nutrient supports your baby's brain and thyroid development. You'll find it in dairy, fish and iodised salt, but if your diet doesn't include much of these (*especially if you're vegan*), a 150mcg supplement is a good idea.

Omega-3 Fatty Acids – particularly DHA (docosahexaenoic acid), play a key role in baby's brain and eye development. The best source? Oily fish, like salmon and sardines. But if fish isn't your thing, don't worry. Look for a prenatal vitamin with at least 200mg of DHA or consider a fish oil or algae-based supplement.

I know this sounds like a LOT to keep track of, but here's the good news – most antenatal vitamins bundle all these nutrients into one tablet. Because let's be real, you're already trying your best not to vomit – the last thing you need is to be choking down 10 different pills each morning.

The Optionals: Nice-to-Haves

There are some vitamins and supplements that get talked about a lot in pregnancy. I call these the 'nice-to-haves'. They can give you an extra boost, but they are not must-haves. And no, I'm not about to tell you to go and create a whole jungle of bottles on your kitchen counter and swallow every pill on the market.

If you're interested in adding an optional supplement, always check with your healthcare provider first. They'll be able to look at what you're already taking and let you know if it's safe to add in something new. A lot of these 'nice-to-haves' are already included in standard pregnancy multivitamins, so it's worth checking the label of what you're currently taking. If it's already covered, you don't need a separate dose.

You can also look at foods that naturally contain these vitamins and minerals – that's always a brilliant option too. And most importantly, don't panic about not getting them. Like the title says, they're nice to have, not essential to have. If you were deficient in any of these areas, your healthcare provider should pick it up and provide the right support.

Calcium – This is key for baby's bone development, but the good news is most women get enough from food. Dairy, fortified plant-based milks, leafy greens and almonds all provide plenty of calcium. But if your diet lacks these, a 500–1000mg supplement might be worth considering. Just one important note – don't take calcium and iron supplements together. They compete for absorption, so it's best to space them a few hours apart for maximum benefit. Your midwife, pharmacist or doctor can give you personalised advice on what will work best for you.

Magnesium – This isn't strictly essential, but if you're dealing with cramps, constipation or insomnia, it can be a game-changer. If you need extra support, 200–400mg daily might help.

B Vitamins – Vitamin B6 is known to help with morning sickness, while B12 is essential if you're vegan. Most prenatal vitamins already include both, but if nausea is taking over your life, you might benefit from an extra 25–50mg of B6 daily.

Zinc – This plays a role in immune function and cell growth, but again – most prenatal vitamins already have you covered. You don't need extra unless you're deficient.

If your diet is varied and balanced, a basic prenatal vitamin with folic acid, vitamin D and iron is usually enough. If you're struggling with nausea or dietary restrictions, supplements like omega-3, magnesium or extra B6 can be helpful. The goal is to support your body – not stress about getting everything perfect. And if your current 'diet' consists of whatever you can keep down, don't panic! Your baby is incredibly good at taking what they need from your body. Just do what you can, and your healthcare providers will keep an eye on your levels as pregnancy progresses.

PREGNANCY AND FOOD SAFETY: THE NO-GOES, THE PRECAUTIONS AND THE MYTHS

Before we get into what's safe and what's not, let's clear something up – pregnancy research is limited, and for good reason. You can't exactly run experiments on pregnant women just to see what's harmful, so most of what we know comes from observational studies, foodborne illness reports and research on non-pregnant people or animals. That said, we do have strong enough evidence to make clear recommendations about what's safe to eat and what's best avoided. So, do I think you'll drop dead if you eat a salmon nigiri? No. Would I advise you to grab raw sushi from a dodgy corner shop where the tuna's been sitting out for who knows how long? Absolutely not. The key here is risk assessment – some foods are definite no-goes, some are fine if handled correctly, and others have been unfairly demonised. Let's break it all down so you can make informed choices without fearmongering.

I'll be honest – this chapter is going to get very science-heavy because I can't stand fear-based advice without real facts to back it up. One thing I love is knowing exactly why something is safe or unsafe – and I want you to have that knowledge too. Science might not be your thing but think of this as arming yourself with information so you can have a safe and confident pregnancy.

What Should You Eat to Support a Healthy Pregnancy?

While it might feel like pregnancy is all about what you can't eat, there's plenty you should eat to give your baby the best start. Your body is working overtime, creating a tiny human inside you, so it needs the right fuel to keep you and your baby healthy. A balanced diet rich in key nutrients can help with everything from foetal development to reducing pregnancy symptoms like fatigue, nausea and constipation.

Start with protein, the building block of your baby's cells, found in lean meats, eggs, fish, beans, lentils and dairy. Iron-rich foods like red meat, spinach and fortified cereals will keep your energy levels up and prevent anaemia. Pairing iron with vitamin C sources (think oranges, bell peppers or strawberries) boosts absorption. Folate-rich foods, such as leafy greens, lentils and oranges, are essential for preventing neural tube defects, while healthy fats like avocado, nuts and salmon support brain development. Whole grains (brown rice, oats, whole-wheat bread) provide fibre to keep digestion moving and help fight pregnancy constipation. Dairy or fortified plant-based alternatives are important for calcium and vitamin D, keeping your baby's bones strong. And let's not forget about hydration – drinking plenty of water will keep your amniotic fluid levels stable, support digestion and help prevent headaches and swelling.

If nausea and food aversions make eating a struggle, don't stress – focus on small, frequent meals packed with as many nutrients as possible. Even if all you can stomach today is toast, your baby will still take what they need from your body. Just aim for a variety of nutrient-rich foods when you can, and don't be afraid to supplement where needed.

Now, let's talk about foods that are absolute no-goes, backed by science. We'll start by looking at what research says, go through which foods to avoid, and I'll also share safe alternatives, so you don't feel like you're missing out.

Foods to Avoid in Pregnancy

Pregnancy alters your immune system, making you more vulnerable to foodborne infections. Some bacteria and parasites, such as toxoplasmosis, listeria and salmonella, can cause severe complications, including miscarriage, stillbirth or serious infections in newborns. While food safety is important for everyone, it becomes even more critical during pregnancy. Below is a guide to some of the main food risks and how to make safer choices.

Raw or Undercooked Meat and Poultry
Consuming raw or undercooked meat increases the risk of exposure to harmful bacteria and parasites.

I'M PREGNANT ... NOW WHAT?

The Research:
- Toxoplasmosis, caused by the *Toxoplasma gondii* parasite, is rare but can have devastating effects on foetal development. A 2019 study found that even mild maternal infections can lead to neurological damage and vision loss in babies.[5]
- Listeria is the bigger concern. Unlike most bacteria, it can grow in refrigerated foods. A UK study found that pregnant women are 20 times more likely to contract listeriosis than the general population.[6]
- Salmonella does not directly harm the baby but can cause severe dehydration and, in rare cases, sepsis.[7]

What to Avoid:
- Rare or undercooked beef, lamb or pork (e.g., rare steaks, carpaccio, steak tartare).
- Raw or undercooked poultry (no pink-in-the-middle chicken or peri-peri medium rare).
- Uncooked cured meats like salami, prosciutto and chorizo (unless cooked).

Safe Options:
- Well-cooked meat (no pink, juices running clear).
- Deli meats only if heated until steaming.

Raw or Partially Cooked Eggs
Eggs are a powerhouse of protein and choline, essential for baby's brain development, but raw eggs can carry

salmonella, which can cause food poisoning and dehydration.

The Research:
- A 2016 UK study found that British Lion Code eggs (stamped with a red lion) have an extremely low risk of salmonella. This led the NHS to update its guidelines, stating that British Lion eggs are safe to eat raw or runny.[8]

What to Avoid:
- Raw eggs from unregulated sources (e.g., backyard chickens).
- Homemade mayonnaise, mousse or hollandaise (unless made with pasteurised eggs).

Safe Options:
- British Lion eggs (runny yolks are fine).
- Pasteurised egg products (used in store-bought mayonnaise).

Soft Cheeses and Unpasteurised Dairy

Soft cheeses may contain listeria, a bacterium that can cross the placenta and harm the baby.

The Research:
- According to the CDC (Centers for Disease Control and Prevention), nearly 25 per cent of pregnancy-

associated cases of listeriosis result in foetal loss or newborn death.[9]

What to Avoid:
- Unpasteurised soft cheeses (brie, camembert, goat's cheese, gorgonzola).
- Raw milk and raw dairy products.

Safe Options:
- Hard cheeses (cheddar, parmesan, Gruyère).
- Soft cheeses if pasteurised (mozzarella, feta, halloumi, cream cheese).

High-Mercury Fish
Mercury is a neurotoxin that can impact your baby's brain and nervous system development.

The Research:
- Higher prenatal mercury exposure (from maternal fish consumption) was associated with measurable effects on cognitive outcomes in children.[10]
- The FDA (Food and Drug Administration) and the WHO (World Health Organization) recommend avoiding high-mercury fish but encourage eating low-mercury fish for essential omega-3 fatty acids.[11]

THE FIRST TRIMESTER

What to Avoid:
- High-mercury fish: shark, swordfish, king mackerel, tilefish.
- Limit tuna to two portions per week.

Safe Alternatives:
- Low-mercury fish: salmon, cod, haddock, sardines, trout.
- Aim for two portions of oily fish per week to boost your baby's brain development.

Liver and High Vitamin A Foods

Too much animal-based vitamin A (retinol) can cause birth defects, especially in early pregnancy.

The Research:
- High intakes of preformed vitamin A (retinol), especially from animal sources or supplements, have been linked to birth defects in humans when consumed in early pregnancy. [12]

What to Avoid:
- Liver, liver pâté, cod liver oil.
- High-dose vitamin A supplements.

Safe Alternatives:
- Plant-based vitamin A (beta-carotene) from carrots, sweet potatoes, spinach.

Controversial Foods (Limited or Conflicting Research)

Caffeine

Some studies suggest high caffeine intake increases the risk of miscarriage or low birth weight, while others say moderate intake is fine.

The Research:
- The NHS and American College of Obstetricians and Gynaecologists (ACOG) recommend limiting caffeine to 200mg per day (about one or two coffees).[13]
- A 2015 meta-analysis found that the risk of miscarriage increased by around 19 per cent for every extra 150mg of caffeine consumed daily.[14]

What to Avoid:
- Excess caffeine (over 200mg daily).
- Energy drinks – some contain too much caffeine and taurine. (Too much taurine, especially when mixed with caffeine, can raise your heart rate and blood pressure, which isn't ideal during pregnancy.)

Safe Amount:
- One small coffee or two cups of tea per day.

THE FIRST TRIMESTER

ILLNESS AND PREGNANCY SYMPTOMS: MEDICATION

Just because you're pregnant doesn't mean you've been magically blessed with immunity from every other illness – unfortunately, you can still get headaches, colds and even the kind of back pain that makes you wonder if you're secretly carrying twins. The good news is that you don't have to suffer in silence.

Paracetamol is your safest bet for pain relief; it's perfectly fine to take. Ibuprofen and aspirin, however, should be avoided, especially in the later months, because your baby doesn't appreciate them. Got a cold or flu? Then you can safely use menthol rubs, saline sprays and honey with lemon. Most decongestants are off the table, but if you're desperate and sound like a blocked drainpipe, your pharmacist might be able to advise on short-term options.

Then there's morning sickness, which doesn't always limit itself to the morning. Ginger, vitamin B6 and acupressure bands might help, but if you're throwing up more than a toddler has tantrums, your doctor can prescribe cyclizine or promethazine to help. Heartburn is another pregnancy classic, and if you're getting that fire-in-your-throat feeling every time you so much as look at food, antacids or acid-reducing meds will be your new best friends – just brace yourself for that thick, chalky texture.

Constipation, as we saw on page 14, is also an unfortunate pregnancy reality because apparently, growing a baby means your digestive system just gives up. If this is your current struggle, and prunes and water aren't cutting it, fibre supplements or stool softeners can help. Stronger laxatives should only be used occasionally, because the cramps they can cause feel a lot like contractions.

For allergies and hay fever, loratadine and cetirizine are safe - so if you're sneezing like a Victorian ghost, you don't have to suffer through it. If you have a UTI, and feel like you're peeing fire, antibiotics such as penicillin and cephalosporins can safely clear it up, but some, like trimethoprim, should be avoided in early pregnancy. Since antibiotics are prescription-only, you don't need to remember this information - your GP should advise on the best course of treatment for you.

The bottom line? Pregnancy doesn't mean you have to suffer through every illness - there are safe options, so always check with your midwife, GP or pharmacist before toughing it out like a martyr.

EXERCISE AND MOVEMENT IN PREGNANCY

This life is all about balance. Pregnancy isn't a nine-month excuse to avoid all movement, nor is it the time to start training for a marathon if your usual workout routine only involves lifting snacks to your mouth.

THE FIRST TRIMESTER

Staying active has huge benefits: it helps with circulation, reduces pregnancy aches and pains, boosts mood, keeps energy levels up, and can even make labour and recovery easier. Exercise also helps lower the risk of gestational diabetes, high blood pressure and excessive weight gain, so it's encouraged. For most women, low-impact, moderate-intensity exercise is ideal. Walking is one of the safest and most effective ways to stay active – it keeps your blood flowing, helps with swelling, and doesn't require any special equipment.

Prenatal yoga and Pilates are great for core strength, flexibility and keeping your pelvic floor in check (which will be very useful when pushing a baby out). Swimming is another brilliant option, especially as your bump grows – floating in water takes the pressure off your joints, making movement feel easier. If you enjoy strength training, light weights and bodyweight exercises are perfectly safe, as long as you're using good form and not overloading yourself. Even if you weren't particularly active before pregnancy, it's never too late to start incorporating gentle movement, which can help with energy levels and reduce common pregnancy discomforts.

While exercise is encouraged, certain activities aren't pregnancy friendly. Anything with a high risk of falling, impact or trauma to the belly should be avoided. Skiing, horse riding, gymnastics and mountain biking might need to be put on hold, as your balance changes throughout pregnancy, making falls more likely. Contact sports like rugby, boxing or martial arts should also be avoided – this is not the time to take a blow to the stomach. Scuba diving is a definite no, as pressure changes can be harmful to foetal development, and hot yoga or any form of excessive heat training should be skipped to prevent overheating. While running isn't off-limits, if you weren't a runner before, now is not the time to start. Stick to lower-impact cardio that won't put excessive strain on your joints.

One of the biggest myths around pregnancy is that exercise can cause a miscarriage. Let's clear that up: exercise does not increase the risk of miscarriage in a healthy pregnancy. The baby is well protected inside the amniotic sac, and normal movement will not dislodge a pregnancy. Unless you have a medical condition where movement is restricted (like placenta praevia or a history of recurrent pregnancy loss), exercise is highly beneficial. That said, it's important to listen to your body and not push yourself too hard. The best way to check if you're exercising at a safe intensity is to use the talk test. If you can still hold a conversation while working out, you're at the right level. If you're gasping for air like you've just run up 10 flights of stairs, it's time to slow down. Pregnancy isn't about setting personal records – it's about moving in a way that keeps you feeling good without overexerting yourself.

Staying active in a way that works for your body will help you feel stronger, more energised and better prepared for the demands of pregnancy, labour and postpartum recovery. So, keep moving, but maybe save the bungee jumping for after birth.

THE FIRST TRIMESTER

EMOTIONAL CARE IN THE FIRST TRIMESTER

No one really prepares you for the emotional whirlwind that hits in the first trimester. Joy, fear, disbelief and exhaustion can all hit once. This section looks at what's happening beneath the surface. Early pregnancy can stir up fears of miscarriage, shift your relationships, challenge your sense of control and bring emotions you didn't even know were sitting there.

FEAR OF MISCARRIAGE – THE ANXIETY NO ONE TALKS ABOUT

This is for those who have never experienced miscarriage but find themselves carrying the weight of its possibility. The fear of the unknown can be just as overwhelming as the pain of loss. If you've walked that path before, your story is different – and it deserves its own space.

The moment you see that positive pregnancy test, a wave of emotions hits – excitement, joy, disbelief and for many, an overwhelming fear of miscarriage. No one prepares you for just how much this fear can take over, how every cramp, every twinge and every moment of feeling 'too normal' can send you spiralling into panic. It's something so many women experience but rarely talk about, because pregnancy is supposed to be all excitement and glowing skin (which is another myth). The truth is, fear of miscarriage is completely normal – especially in the first trimester, when everything feels uncertain and out of your control. You're suddenly hyper-aware of every symptom (or lack of symptoms), googling things like 'does a drop in nausea mean miscarriage?' at 2 a.m. and analysing your toilet paper like a forensic investigator. It's exhausting and yet it's rarely discussed openly.

What's Actually in Your Control?

The hardest part of early pregnancy is accepting that most miscarriages happen due to chromosomal issues or developmental problems that we have no power over. It's not because you lifted something heavy, didn't eat enough vegetables or walked too fast up the stairs. It's not because you had sex or because you stressed too much at work. Most miscarriages happen for reasons that are completely beyond your control, and no amount of anxiety will change the outcome. That doesn't mean your feelings aren't valid – it just means that blaming yourself won't change the reality.

How to Cope with the Fear

It's easy to say, 'Just relax,' but let's be real – if it were that simple, anxiety would not exist. Instead of trying to ignore the fear, acknowledge it. Talk to someone you trust, whether it's your partner, a friend or your midwife. Focus on what you can control – taking your prenatal vitamins, staying hydrated, getting enough rest – but don't obsess over every little thing.

Distractions help, too. Find things that make you feel good, whether it's a light walk, watching a favourite show or diving into a good book. If you've had a miscarriage before, the anxiety can be even more intense. Every ache and cramp can feel like history repeating itself. In that case, asking for extra reassurance from your midwife or doctor isn't being dramatic – it's advocating for your mental well-being. Some women find early scans helpful, while others feel that they just fuel the anxiety more. Do what feels right for you.

The Reality Check – Most Pregnancies Are Healthy

Here's something no one tells you when you're spiralling with worry: most pregnancies are completely fine. By the time you see a heartbeat on an early scan, the risk of miscarriage drops significantly. And once you hit the second trimester, the odds are heavily in your favour. But because so many of us are wired to fear the worst, it's easy to focus on the stories of loss rather than the millions of healthy pregnancies happening every day. It's okay to be scared. It's okay to feel anxious. But don't let the fear steal your joy. You are pregnant *right now*. And right now, that's enough.

HOW PREGNANCY CHANGES YOUR RELATIONSHIPS – PARTNER, FAMILY AND FRIENDS

Pregnancy doesn't just change your body; it also changes your relationships in ways you might not have expected.

I'M PREGNANT ... NOW WHAT?

Some relationships grow stronger, some become more strained, and some don't change at all, which can be just as frustrating. Whether it's your partner, your parents or even your closest friends, suddenly everyone has opinions about your pregnancy, and sometimes, those opinions come with big emotions. One minute, you're getting unconditional support; the next, you're dealing with unsolicited advice, emotional distance or family members acting like they're the ones having the baby. While some of these changes bring people closer, others might seriously test your patience.

If you have a partner, you might assume that because you're pregnant together, you'll be experiencing everything the same way. The reality? Pregnancy hits differently for the person carrying the baby. You feel every symptom, every kick, every hormonal shift. Your partner, on the other hand, is watching from the sidelines, trying to figure out what their role is in all of this. Some partners jump in immediately, cooking, rubbing your feet and reading every pregnancy book like their life depends on it. Others struggle, either because they're overwhelmed, nervous or just don't feel connected to the pregnancy yet. Unlike you, they don't have the constant physical reminder that a baby is coming, which can make them seem a little detached. This doesn't mean they don't care; it just means their experience of pregnancy is completely different.

You might also notice new tensions in your relationship. Maybe you're feeling more emotional and need reassurance, while your partner thinks they're helping by focusing on practical things like budgeting and logistics. Maybe your libido has disappeared, and they don't know what to do with that information. Or maybe you're beyond irritated that they can sleep through the night while you're up peeing for the fifth time. The key to navigating all of this? Communication. Be honest about how you're feeling, even if it's completely irrational (*pregnancy hormones are powerful*). Encourage them to ask questions, learn about what's happening, and get involved in ways that feel meaningful to both of you.

And what about your parents? For some, your pregnancy is the best news ever - they can't wait to become grandparents and are already reminiscing about their own pregnancy stories (even though medical advice has changed a lot since then). For others, your pregnancy might bring up complicated emotions, especially if they have unresolved feelings about their own parenting journey. Some parents become overly involved, others seem distant and sometimes, neither reaction has anything to do with you. If they're supportive, amazing! But if they start overstepping by telling you how to raise your child, making comments about your body or treating your pregnancy like a community project, it's okay to set boundaries. You are not obligated to listen to every single piece of advice. And if they're distant, try not to take it personally. Not everyone knows how to show up in the way you might need, so focus on building your own village: friends, loved ones or fellow parents who make you feel seen and supported.

I'M PREGNANT ... NOW WHAT?

Friendships can shift during pregnancy, especially if your friends are in a different stage of life. Some will be excited, supportive and involved in your journey. Others may pull away, either because they don't relate to your new reality or assume you are too busy to hang out. It can be hard when friendships change, but it's also a chance to see which ones truly matter.

And this is something a lot of people feel. Remember, most of your friends have never experienced their friendship with you as a pregnant woman. You are learning, and so are they. Some people are emotionally intelligent enough to adapt, while others may struggle to make that shift. That doesn't always mean the friendship is over – it just means it might look different for a while.

It also helps to see the other side. Pregnancy opens up space for new friendships too. Friendships thrive on relatability, and you may find that you naturally connect with other pregnant women at antenatal classes or baby groups. One of my closest friends, Dami, since having her baby, has built new friendships with other mums. Did I think she needed new friends? Maybe, maybe not. But she has them now, and they're off doing baby dates and playdates. And for now, I don't have a baby to bring, and it's just not my vibe. That's not a friendship I would join in on right now, so those playdates are not ones I would attend.

And then there are the day-to-day changes too. The phone calls we used to have that once flowed with ease now often come with a background chorus of 'Mum, Mum, Mum'

THE FIRST TRIMESTER

500 times. Do our conversations go as smoothly? Absolutely not. But we've learned to adjust, and that adjustment has kept the friendship strong. Not everyone will be able to do that though, and that's okay. Pregnancy and motherhood bring an element of selflessness that only motherhood really teaches you. When someone has not had to experience that, they might find it harder to relate. That's where empathy comes in because you don't have to go through something yourself to at least try to understand it. Some friends will be able to show that, and some won't, because everyone is different. But what I will say is this: don't go into pregnancy already expecting your friendships to break. That mindset can become a self-fulfilling prophecy.

At the same time, you may be able to maintain older friendships, just in a new way. When Dami was pregnant, our friendship definitely changed. We're still very close, but we no longer see each other every other day. Instead, we meet up once every few months, usually for a long walk, and that works beautifully for us. Not everyone can make that adjustment, but it showed me that friendships can evolve rather than end.

My best advice is to speak up. Tell your friends what you need, even if you're not sure yet. Say you're figuring it out. That honesty gives your friendship a chance to adjust alongside you. What doesn't help is going into pregnancy expecting friendships to stay exactly the same or setting such high expectations that no one can meet them. Be considerate too – this is new territory for them as much as it is for you. Pregnancy is a huge life shift, and relationships will evolve with it: some will grow stronger, some will become more challenging, and some will fade away altogether. The best thing you can do is be clear about your needs, set boundaries and accept that not everyone will get it – and that's okay. The people who truly care will adjust, just as you are adjusting to this new chapter of your life.

MOOD SWINGS AND EMOTIONS: DEALING WITH HORMONAL SHIFTS

One minute you're crying at a puppy video, the next you're irrationally furious because someone *breathed too loudly* near you. Pregnancy mood swings are not for the weak, and if you're feeling emotionally unhinged, just know you're not alone. Your hormones are rising at record-breaking speeds, your body is working overtime to grow a human, and your brain is trying to process the fact that life is about to change forever. It's a *lot*. Pregnancy mood swings are mainly driven by hormonal shifts, particularly oestrogen and progesterone, which can affect neurotransmitters in your brain (the chemicals responsible for mood regulation). Throw in exhaustion, nausea and the occasional existential crisis about becoming a parent, and it's no wonder you feel like an emotional rollercoaster. It's completely normal, but that doesn't mean it's easy.

First things first: don't beat yourself up for feeling *too much*. Whether you're crying over spilt milk (literally) or snapping at your partner for existing too loudly, remind yourself that this is temporary and completely normal. Your body is going through massive changes, and your emotions are just keeping up. Lack of sleep and hunger make everything worse. If you've ever been 'hangry' before pregnancy, just multiply that feeling by 10 and add hormones into the mix. Eating regularly and getting enough rest won't erase the mood swings, but they can help stop you from hitting emotional rock bottom over something minor. Always keep snacks nearby – trust me on this one.

Exercise might be the last thing you want to do when you're feeling moody, but it can actually help regulate your emotions. Even a short walk or some gentle stretching can boost your mood by increasing endorphins (your brain's 'happy' chemicals).

If your partner, friends or family are walking on eggshells around you, it's probably because they don't understand what's happening in your head. Tell them how you're feeling, even if it sounds irrational. Sometimes, just saying, 'I don't know why I'm upset, but I need support' is enough to keep small tensions from turning into full-blown arguments. Some days, nothing will help except curling up in bed with snacks and your favourite Netflix show. Have a plan for when you're feeling emotionally drained, whether it's watching a comfort movie, listening to music, journalling or calling a friend. Give yourself grace. Mood swings are normal, but if your sadness, anxiety or irritability start feeling overwhelming or persistent, it's important to reach out for help. Perinatal depression and anxiety are real, and you don't have to suffer in silence. If you're feeling consistently low, speak to your midwife or doctor – they're there to support you, not judge you.

Pregnancy emotions are unpredictable, and some days, you might not even recognise yourself. That's okay. Your body is doing something incredible, and your mind is just trying to keep up. So, whether you're crying over an advert, laughing uncontrollably at something that isn't funny or needing space from everyone, just go with it. Mood swings are temporary, but the strength you're building through this process? That will stay with you long after pregnancy.

PREGNANCY PLANNING: THE DECISIONS NO ONE TALKS ABOUT

Pregnancy isn't just about growing a tiny human – it comes with a whole load of decisions, plans and *logistics*. From choosing the right healthcare provider to figuring out when to tell your boss, sorting your finances and resisting the urge to buy every baby gadget in sight, this section is here to help you make informed, stress-free choices. Whether you're debating between government-funded and private healthcare, wondering how to break the news to your employer or trying to budget for a baby without going broke, I've got you covered. Think of this as your practical guide to tackling the behind-the-scenes prep so you can focus on the exciting, if sometimes chaotic, journey ahead.

THE FIRST TRIMESTER

CHOOSING A HEALTHCARE PROVIDER: NHS VS. PRIVATE

One of the biggest decisions you'll make in pregnancy is choosing your healthcare provider. In the UK, you have two main options: the NHS or private care. There's no one-size-fits-all answer because your experience isn't just about the hospital or clinic you choose – it's about the individuals who care for you.

People often ask me, 'What's the best hospital to give birth in?' And my honest answer is that there isn't one. You could go to the most highly rated hospital with glowing reviews and still have a terrible experience. On the flip side, you could go to a hospital that people swear they'd never return to and meet midwives who provide the most incredible care.

Here's the thing about online reviews: they're often written by people who had a bad experience. Those who had a great experience? They're more likely to show their gratitude with a box of chocolates for the staff than a five-star review. This means hospital ratings don't always reflect the quality of care you might receive. So, my advice is to start with what's convenient. Choose a hospital near you. If you have a bad experience, you can always move. But don't drive yourself mad searching for the 'perfect' place, because ultimately, it's about the care you receive, not the building you're in.

Now, let's talk about the NHS versus private care. I'm not here to tell you which one to choose, as this decision is deeply personal and depends on your needs and circumstances. If you want one-on-one care, luxurious surroundings and a more tailored experience, private care might be for you. You'll get more time with your provider, more personalised attention and fewer rushed appointments. But this comes at a literal cost.

If private care isn't financially feasible, the NHS is a solid option. The NHS has seen everything. No matter what you're experiencing, there's a midwife or doctor who has handled it before. You're not likely to surprise them. And while NHS resources can sometimes be stretched, the knowledge and expertise within the system are second to none.

I've worked in both the NHS and the private sector, and let me tell you, the difference is wild. The first time I realised I was in a whole different world in private care? The coffee machine. That machine was gorgeous – the kind that makes you feel like you've stepped into a high-end café rather than a hospital. That's when I knew: I was no longer with the NHS.

Private care is luxury care. The women are pampered. Everything can be done for them. I remember how we would change the babies' nappies like we were on a concierge service. Meanwhile, in the NHS? Yeah, that's not happening. It's not because the midwives don't care, but because they literally don't have the time. In the NHS, midwives are often fighting for their lives just to provide basic care. They're overstretched, underfunded and working within a system that demands more than it gives. But here's

THE FIRST TRIMESTER

what I need you to understand: just because NHS midwives are overworked doesn't mean they don't care. They care deeply.

So, should you go private or NHS? That depends on you. If you want luxury, if you want someone fluffing your pillows and if you have the budget, go private. If private care is not within your means, don't feel like you're signing up for horror stories by going NHS. NHS midwives are some of the most skilled and experienced professionals out there. Do your research. Weigh up what your money allows. But what I never want anyone to feel is that choosing the NHS means they're automatically going to receive sub-standard care. Your experience will depend on the midwives looking after you, and trust me, a lot of NHS midwives will do everything they can, even when the system makes it hard for them.

THE IMPORTANCE OF A JUST IN CASE (JIC) FUND

Every time I feel someone is disrespecting me, the first thing I ask myself is, 'Am I being unreasonable?' and if the answer is no, I make sure I have the resources to remove myself from the situation. That's the kind of power I want you to have over your pregnancy care, so that if you ever feel dismissed or unheard you're not just stuck. If there's one feeling I *hate*, it's helplessness. I don't want that for you. I never want you to be in a situation where you feel like you have no options, especially when it comes to your care. That's why I always tell my mamas, especially if opting for the NHS: *start a JIC fund.*

I know private care isn't an option for everyone, but having *some* money set aside means that if NHS appointments are booked up or they don't think your concern is urgent, you can just go and pay for a private scan or appointment *without stress.* It's not about replacing NHS care – it's about making sure you're never at the mercy of a stretched system with no backup plan, or needing extra tests you didn't account for and feeling panicked. So, my advice? Plan for the unexpected. Even if you never need it, knowing you *could* do something about a situation if you had to offers priceless peace of mind.

CHOOSING THE RIGHT HOSPITAL FOR YOU

Regardless of whether you go down the NHS or private route, there are a few key things you should consider before choosing a hospital for your maternity care. First, think about location and accessibility. Is the hospital close enough for you to get there quickly in labour, and what are the parking or transport options like for you and your birth partner? Next, look into the type of care available. Does the hospital have a midwifery-led unit for a more natural birth experience, or is it consultant-led with facilities for higher-risk pregnancies? If a water birth is something you'd like, check if they have birthing pools available.

Consider the hospital's policies and facilities, such as whether partners can stay overnight, if epidurals are available 24/7, and what kind of postnatal support they offer, including breastfeeding help and mental health care. It's also worth asking about birth preferences, like their approach to C-sections, inductions, delayed cord clamping and immediate skin-to-skin contact.

If you're weighing up NHS versus private care, find out whether the hospital offers private maternity services and what's included, such as one-to-one midwifery care or private rooms. Lastly, speak to people who have given birth there, check real-life experiences and, if possible, visit the hospital or take a virtual tour, because while online reviews can give some insight, nothing beats trusting your instincts.

WORK AND PREGNANCY: WHEN AND HOW TO TELL YOUR EMPLOYER

Deciding when to tell your employer about your pregnancy is personal, and there's no one-size-fits-all answer. It depends on you, your symptoms, your job and how you feel about sharing the news. The first trimester, as we've already discussed, can be struggle central. If you're managing fine and prefer to keep things quiet, there's no rush. But if you're battling constant nausea, exhaustion that makes getting through the workday feel like a full marathon, or needing to disappear for frequent toilet breaks, telling your employer sooner might make things easier. The instinct to keep it private, especially with the fear of miscarriage, is completely understandable – but if symptoms are making work unbearable, it's worth weighing up whether having that conversation earlier would actually help.

The type of work you do also plays a huge role in when you should break the news. If your job mostly involves sitting at a desk answering emails, you might not feel any urgency, but if your job is physically demanding, involves exposure to chemicals, or – let's say – bungee jumping for a living, then you need to let your employer know straight away. Certain jobs pose risks to pregnancy, and employers have a legal obligation to make adjustments for you. Healthcare workers, those in construction, hospitality or any role that requires long hours on their feet should consider telling their employer earlier to ensure safety measures are in place.

Legally, in the UK, you're not required to tell your employer you're pregnant until 15 weeks before your due date, which is around 25 weeks pregnant. However, that doesn't mean you should wait that long, especially if your job needs adjustments. Once you inform your employer, they're required to carry out a risk assessment, give you time off for antenatal appointments and ensure you aren't discriminated against due to your pregnancy. You are not asking for permission to be pregnant – you are informing them of a fact, and they are legally required to support you.

When it comes to actually breaking the news, think about how you want to approach it. Some people prefer a formal email, while others opt for a face-to-face conversation. Consider your manager's personality, your company's work culture and your own comfort level. No matter how you do it, be clear and confident. Once the news is out, you might need to navigate work differently. Pregnancy can be unpredictable; some days you'll feel fine, other days you'll be struggling to keep your eyes open before lunch. If your workplace allows for flexible hours, remote work or adjusted duties, it might be worth discussing these options. And if you ever feel unsupported or that your employer is treating you unfairly because of your pregnancy, remember: employment law is on your side.

PLANNING YOUR MATERNITY LEAVE: RIGHTS, TIMEFRAMES AND PAPERWORK

Once you do decide to share the news with your employer, there are a few important steps to take when it comes to planning your maternity leave. You'll need to confirm in writing that you're pregnant, your due date, and when you'd like your maternity leave to start – by the same 25-week point mentioned earlier. Your midwife will give you a MATB1 form at around 20 weeks, which is the official certificate that confirms your due date. Hand that to your employer, and that's the paperwork side sorted.

Now, I'm not going to go into exact figures on how much maternity pay you're entitled to because these things change all the time and depend heavily on your job, your contract and your circumstances. What I *will* say is: find out as soon as possible what your workplace offers. Some companies are very generous; others stick to the legal minimum – so get clarity early so you can plan properly.

The main thing is to know your timeline, hand in your MATB1 and get clear on what support you'll actually receive so you can focus less on paperwork and more on preparing for your baby.

For My Self-Employed Mamas

Being self-employed while pregnant is a whole different experience. There's no HR department, no automatic paid maternity leave and no team to pick up the slack when pregnancy fatigue hits. Everything falls on you, which means planning ahead is essential. The good news is that self-employment comes with flexibility, but the challenge is ensuring you have financial security while you navigate pregnancy and time off. One of the first things to look into is financial support.

In the UK, self-employed women may be eligible for Maternity Allowance, a government benefit designed for those who don't qualify for Statutory Maternity Pay. If you've been paying Class 2 National Insurance contributions, you could receive payments for up to 39 weeks. It's worth checking eligibility early so you know what to expect. Saving ahead of time is also crucial if your income fluctuates. If possible, start putting money aside during pregnancy so you have a financial cushion when you need to slow down or take maternity leave.

THE FIRST TRIMESTER

Managing workload is another major factor. Pregnancy might not instantly affect your ability to work, but as it progresses, exhaustion, nausea and general discomfort can make keeping up with deadlines feel impossible. If your work involves client-based services or running a business, consider restructuring your workload early. Can you batch content? Automate systems? Reduce client load? Preparing for this in advance will save you from unnecessary stress later. If outsourcing is an option, whether that's hiring a virtual assistant or bringing in temporary help, it's worth considering.

Communication is also key. If you work with clients or customers, let them know your availability as your due date approaches. Set clear boundaries about response times and expected delays in service. If your business allows for passive income, this could be a game-changer. Thinking ahead about how you can keep income flowing without actively working will give you more peace of mind.

For My Mamas Who Aren't Working

Finding out you're pregnant when you're unemployed can feel overwhelming, especially if money is already tight, but there are options and support available. Financially, there are benefits that can help, including Universal Credit, or Employment and Support Allowance, if pregnancy affects your ability to work. If it's your first baby and you're on a low income, you might also be eligible for the Sure Start Maternity Grant, a one-off £500 payment to help with baby costs. Even if you haven't worked recently, you might still qualify for Maternity Allowance based on past earnings. It's worth checking what you're entitled to early on so you can plan accordingly.

If you're considering work during pregnancy but need flexibility, remote jobs, freelancing or part-time work might be worth exploring. There are plenty of online platforms where you can find freelance gigs in writing, virtual assistance, customer service and more. If finding a job right now isn't realistic, you might want to explore free or low-cost training courses. Some local councils, charities or online platforms offer courses that could help if you're thinking about future employment. Volunteering can also be a way to gain experience while keeping structure in your routine.

One of the biggest struggles of being unemployed during pregnancy is the emotional toll. It's easy to feel like you should be doing more, but pregnancy is already a huge life change. Your worth is not defined by a paycheque or job title. If you're feeling isolated, try connecting with other pregnant women through antenatal classes, online communities or local support groups. Having a support system can make a huge difference in how you experience pregnancy.

Whether you're employed, self-employed or not working at all, pregnancy brings up a lot of financial and emotional considerations. The key is to plan ahead, explore your options, and make the best decision for your situation. Work is important, but so is your health. As you already know by now, pregnancy is a full-time job in itself. You deserve to feel supported, no matter your employment status.

WHAT TO START BUYING (AND WHAT NOT TO YET): AVOIDING UNNECESSARY EARLY PURCHASES

One of the biggest traps pregnant women fall into is the idea that the more they buy, the better a mother they will be. The baby product industry thrives off this belief, convincing expectant parents that they need *everything* before the baby even arrives. From endless lists of 'must-haves' to beautifully marketed, overpriced products, brands know exactly how to prey on that *new mum anxiety*. They sell you this dream that if you don't have the latest baby gadget, you're somehow already failing before the baby is even born. But let's be real – half of this stuff is *not* essential.

The truth is that newborns need very little in the beginning. They don't care about designer prams, aesthetic nurseries or the latest self-rocking bassinet. They care about warmth, food and being close to you. Yet, the moment you announce your pregnancy, you're bombarded with marketing that makes it seem like you need to spend thousands just to be a 'prepared' mum – and it works because pregnancy comes with a lot of uncertainty, and shopping feels like *control*. You might not know what birth will be like, but you can choose the 'best' pram. You might not know if breastfeeding will work out, but you can have the top-rated breast pump *just in case*. And before you know it, you've spent a fortune on things you might never even use.

WHAT TO BUY IN THE FIRST TRIMESTER (AND WHAT CAN WAIT)

The first trimester is overwhelming enough without feeling like you need to start shopping immediately. The truth? There isn't a *long* list of things you need to buy at this stage. The baby isn't arriving tomorrow, and you've got time. Pregnancy is a marathon, not a sprint. There are a few things worth considering early on, not necessarily for the baby, but for *you*. This stage of pregnancy can be rough, and anything that makes it more manageable is worth investing in.

Comfortable clothing is a good start. If you're feeling bloated and sick, the last thing you need is tight waistbands digging into you. You don't necessarily need maternity clothes yet, but a couple of stretchy leggings or looser-fitting outfits can make all the difference.

If nausea is hitting hard, stock up on whatever helps. Whether that's ginger biscuits, travel sickness bands or electrolyte drinks, this is the time to find what works for *your* body.

A pregnancy pillow might not feel like a priority now, but as your body starts changing, having extra support when you sleep can be a game-changer.

One thing that's definitely worth buying early is a good prenatal vitamin. This isn't about marketing – as we discussed

THE FIRST TRIMESTER

earlier (see page 28) this is genuinely one of the few 'must-haves' that matter. To recap: folic acid and vitamin D are essential in early pregnancy, and if your nausea is making it hard to eat well, a prenatal vitamin can help cover any nutritional gaps.

At this stage, there's no rush to start buying for the baby. Later in the book, we'll get into what's actually worth buying for labour, postpartum and newborn essentials. For now, the focus should be on making *you* feel as comfortable and supported as possible.

TO ANNOUNCE OR NOT TO ANNOUNCE . . . THAT IS THE QUESTION

Now listen – I've said it before, and I'll say it again: **you don't need to announce your pregnancy**. Not to your followers, not to your colleagues, not even to your aunty with the loudest mouth in the family WhatsApp group. You can keep it to yourself for as long as you like. That choice is yours – full stop. But if you *do* want to tell people, well . . . let's get into the fun part.

See, this is the bit I absolutely love. This is the cute part. The part where you get to share your joy with the world on your terms, in your own way. And some of the creative ways people choose to announce their pregnancy? Gorgeous. Literally had me in tears one moment and grinning like a proud aunty the next. But before we get into all the cute ideas, let me say this: you can't hide forever.

I'M PREGNANT ... NOW WHAT?

Pregnancy is one of those things that becomes harder and harder to hide. Even if you decide not to announce it, the world has a weird way of figuring it out. You go quiet on social media for a few weeks, and suddenly the comments start rolling in: 'Haven't seen her in a while ...' 'She's glowing differently ...' Or my personal favourite: 'This one is pregnant. I can feel it in my spirit.'

I don't know what sixth sense people develop when it comes to pregnancy, but honestly, they know. So even if you don't post a thing, just know that some people will clock it regardless. But when *you* decide to share it (if ever!), you get to set the tone.

If you are thinking of announcing your pregnancy, here are some cute, funny, emotional and all-around iconic ways people do it . . .

1. **The Hug-and-Scan Drop (Slow-Mo Edition)**
   You and your partner are locked in an emotional embrace, soft music playing in the background, maybe a little blurry lens action . . . and then bam! – the scan photo drops in slow motion. Listen. Every time I see this, I have to pause and take it in. It's cinematic. It's sweet. It's so clean.
2. **The Cupcake Reveal**
   A bite into a cupcake and – surprise! – there's a pink or blue filling or a tiny scan pic inside. Sometimes it's

THE FIRST TRIMESTER

the icing that says, 'Baby Coming Soon'. Either way, it's adorable. Sweet-tooth girlies, this one's for you.

3. **The 'Intimate' Video**

   I love this one because it's full of emotion – happy tears, soft lighting, raw reactions to finding out. But let's be honest, once you've uploaded it to everyone who follows you on Instagram, it's not that intimate any more. Still cute though. Still crying in the comments.

4. **Pet Participation**

   If you've got a dog, cat or even a guinea pig, throw them a little sign: 'Big Brother in Training' or 'Guard Dog on Duty – Baby Incoming'. Every time I see this, I melt.

5. **Matching Tees or Hoodies**

   You and your partner in T-shirts that say 'Mum' and 'Dad' or 'Bun in the Oven' and 'Oven Operator'. Cheesy? Maybe. But honestly, I eat it up every time.

6. **The Film Poster Reveal**

   Create a movie poster: 'Coming Soon: Baby [Surname]' with a due date and dramatic tagline. I've seen people go all out with this – cinematic fonts, mood lighting and even ratings like 'Rated P for Parent'.

7. **Voice Note or Audio Reveal**

   Record the sound of your baby's heartbeat and overlay it on a black screen with the words: 'Our little secret's got a heartbeat'. It's minimalist but powerful. Straight chills.

8. Big Sibling Drop

   If this isn't your first baby, older siblings are the perfect way to make the announcement. A shirt that says, 'Promoted to Big Sister' or a picture of them holding the scan like, 'Can't wait to meet you!' – heart, melted.

9. Caption-Only Soft Drop

   You post a regular pic – maybe you in a cute outfit, not a bump in sight – but the caption says, 'Currently growing organs'. And just like that, chaos in the comments. People zooming in, reading between the lines.

Also, Let's Acknowledge This . . .

Now, one thing I do want to say, because it's important, is that in some cultures, pregnancy is something you keep to yourself. It's sacred. It's intimate. It stays within the family. And some religions even speak about the evil eye, this idea that not everyone watching is watching with love, so it's best not to put everything out there. And that's absolutely valid.

You're allowed to protect your peace. You're allowed to keep your pregnancy close. You're allowed to say, 'Actually, this is just for us.' But I also want you to know that it doesn't mean you can't still capture those beautiful moments. You can still do the dramatic photo shoot. The dreamy sunset gown. The handwritten letter to your unborn baby. You can still have your main character moment – you don't have to share it anywhere.

Make the memory anyway.

UNIQUE JOURNEYS FOR THE FIRST TRIMESTER

This section talks about pregnancy after loss, specifically what it can feel like in the first trimester if you've had a miscarriage or another kind of loss. I want to say from the start: *you don't have to read this right now.* You might be someone who *has* experienced loss and would rather not revisit it in this moment – and that's completely okay. You might *not* have experienced loss, but know your mind has a tendency to spiral and imagine the worst – that's also okay. We'll also discuss hyperemesis gravidarum and include a real story that touches on pregnancy termination due to severe illness. Please read at your own pace – this is a space for honesty and support, but it's only safe if you feel ready. Other sections cover different experiences, like unexpected or accidental pregnancies, finding out you're carrying twins or multiples, surrogacy or gestational carrier pregnancy, pregnancy in a larger or older body (including fatphobia and ageism in healthcare), and pregnancy after fertility treatments – adjusting to 'normal' after a medicalised journey. You can choose what feels right for you to read.

I'M PREGNANT ... NOW WHAT?

This book is big on one thing: taking in only the information you can handle. You are allowed to protect your peace. Come back to this or any other section later if you want to, or skip it entirely. Either way, you are still doing what you need to do for you, and that is more than enough.

PREGNANCY AFTER LOSS – NAVIGATING EMOTIONS IN THE FIRST TRIMESTER

This is a section I was nervous to write.

I like to know what I'm trying to do before I start writing. I like knowing what I hope you'll feel when you read my words. But with this section, there's no clear path. No guaranteed outcome. This is one of those topics where even the most carefully chosen words might fall short. And honestly, I think that's what makes it important to write. If you're reading this and you've been pregnant before, only to lose that pregnancy, I want to start by saying this: I see you. I might not say 'sorry' in the traditional way, because it's not just about pity. It's more like an ache I feel on your behalf. A knowing. A recognition that you've been robbed of something that should have been yours, freely: the blissful ignorance of early pregnancy.

You were supposed to get to feel joy without the weight. You were supposed to just be pregnant. But now you carry something else too. You carry memory, and fear and the strange in-between space of hope and hesitation. And that's not fair. Your fear is fast. It jumps ahead of logic, it overrides

THE FIRST TRIMESTER

reassurance. You can be mid-conversation or in the middle of Tesco, and suddenly your chest drops. Your mind scrambles to find what's wrong, and then you remember. Oh. It's the fear again. That subtle but sharp panic. It lives under your skin now. You never invited it, but here it is.

Maybe people tell you to 'think positive' or 'don't stress'. But that's the thing – they don't get it. You *are* thinking positive. You're still here, still pregnant, still reading this, despite everything. That *is* hope. It's just a version of hope that's been through something. It's cautious, maybe quieter but it's no less real.

This space is not to fix anything. I won't pretend to have a magic line that will erase the worry. Because even if I did, it might only last until the next cramp or quiet moment when your mind starts spinning again. But I can offer you this: a space where your feelings aren't 'too much'. Where you're not being dramatic or negative or ungrateful. You're just human. A human who's been through something difficult, now trying to move forward while still holding that past.

And maybe that's the real strength in this trimester for you – not pretending everything's okay but learning how to carry your fear and your hope in the same hand.

This is Sam's story. She's not only my colleague but also my friend. She's a midwife who experienced five miscarriages before going on to have a baby. You would think that being surrounded by other midwives would mean she was always held in the right words, but loss has a way of making people panic. Even colleagues who knew better still said things that cut deep, like, 'maybe you work too hard' or 'you should be grateful it's early'. That is the thing about loss – it makes people uncomfortable, and often they reach for words that miss the mark.

But Sam also remembered the one moment when words landed. A colleague took her hands and said, 'Delay is not denial.' She told me it was the only thing anyone ever said that truly comforted her. For her, those words became an anchor. For you, it might be something else – maybe a prayer, maybe an affirmation, maybe a simple reminder that says, *I am pregnant today, and that is enough.* If faith is part of your life, this may be the time to lean on it, to let scriptures or mantras or prayers carry you when your own words run out.

Sam's story shows that there is no single right way through pregnancy after loss. Every experience is different. And just as important as leaning on affirmations is allowing yourself to be honest: if the joy or the fearlessness isn't there, you don't have to pretend that it is. If the excitement comes, let it. If the fear comes, name it. Both can exist side by side, and both are real.

It can also help to have someone close to you who can advocate for you, whether that's your partner, a family member or a trusted friend. There may be times when you don't feel able to speak for yourself, and that's okay. Someone else can step in to help steer off unwanted or unwelcome advice, so you don't have to carry that weight on your own.

Sam's story is a reminder that you don't have to be fixed, and you don't need to have all the answers. Even saying 'I don't know what I want right now' is enough. Sometimes, just admitting that is the bravest step of all.

ACCIDENTAL PREGNANCY – DEALING WITH UNEXPECTED FEELINGS

Planned pregnancies already come with an overload of emotions, let alone one you didn't plan. Maybe the pull-out method didn't work this time (even though it's not really meant to work), or the implant failed. Maybe you missed a pill. Maybe you didn't even realise your body was ovulating again. Maybe you did everything 'right' and still ended up staring at two lines, wondering how and why *now*?

Whatever happened, you're pregnant.

And maybe, just maybe, you're not even sure if you're going ahead with it. That's okay too. I can only assume you might be continuing if you're reading this chapter but let me tell you now: I stopped assuming anything after I once told a patient her mum was outside, and it turned out to be her wife. (In my defence, they looked alike.)

So, let's talk about the emotions that come when a pregnancy wasn't part of the plan. For some, it's a first pregnancy and your mind is spinning with shock, fear – maybe even guilt for not feeling instantly excited. You're trying to figure out what this means for your future, your finances, your body, your mental health. It's like standing still while life speeds up around you.

I'M PREGNANT ... NOW WHAT?

But for others, this surprise comes just after having a baby. You're still recovering physically, mentally and emotionally. You might still be bleeding. You're breastfeeding. You haven't slept properly in weeks. And now, somehow, you're pregnant again. Two under two. Or in some cases ... two under *one*. Yes, it happens. A lot more than people talk about.

And this type of unplanned pregnancy brings its own storm of feelings. The panic isn't always about *whether* you want another child – it's more about *how* you're going to survive it. Your body hasn't finished healing, your baby is still in arms, and now you're being asked to do it all again.

You might feel guilty, exhausted, resentful, numb or strangely calm. You might have cried. You might have laughed because it was so ridiculous you didn't know what else to do. It's okay. All of that is okay.

Let's be real – parenting is already full-on. Being pregnant while still learning how to parent a small baby? That's next level. So, if you're feeling overwhelmed, confused or unsure, let me remind you: you're not broken, and you're not alone.

Take a breath. Let's go back to the basics. Talk to someone. Say the hard things out loud: the fears, the questions, the feelings you're not proud of. Get them out of your head and into a space where they can be heard and held with compassion. Look at your reality with kindness. What's working? What needs adjusting? Do you have support? Do you need to ask for more? Are there systems,

THE FIRST TRIMESTER

routines or boundaries you can begin to explore now, even if they're just tiny ones?

Most importantly, give yourself permission to feel it all. This pregnancy might not have started with joy. That doesn't mean it can't become meaningful. And if you're still in the place of figuring out what this means for you, take your time. Pregnancy doesn't mean certainty – and that's okay too. There's no 'right' reaction to a surprise pregnancy. You are doing something incredibly human right now: navigating the unexpected. And whether it is your first baby, or you're holding one while carrying another, you deserve support, softness and space to figure it all out.

And if this is your first pregnancy and you're reading all of this thinking, *Oh hell no, I am not doing a back-to-back pregnancy*, then let me gently (and firmly) say: start thinking about contraception now. Because one thing that's not spoken about enough is just how fertile you can be after giving birth (see page 277).

TWIN OR MULTIPLE PREGNANCY – WHEN YOU LEAVE THE SCAN WITH DOUBLE (OR TRIPLE) NEWS

You think you're just going in for a routine scan. Maybe you're feeling a little nervous, maybe even a little excited. You're hoping to hear that everything looks okay. You lie down, they squirt the gel, press the probe and then the sonographer pauses. Not because anything's wrong . . . but because there's more than *one*. More than one head. More than one heartbeat. More than one *everything*. You're having twins. Or triplets. Or more.

Suddenly, everything changes. Your brain does somersaults before your body even reacts. For a lot of people, it's pure shock. The kind where your mouth smiles but your soul is in the corner doing deep breathing. It's not that you're not happy – it's just that you *weren't ready* for this kind of plot twist.

Maybe you're thinking about space. About money. About childcare. About your car. About your sanity. Maybe you're calculating how many nappies that actually means in a week. Maybe you're wondering if your body can *actually* do this – and yes, it can – but it will ask a lot of you. Twin and multiple pregnancies hit different in the first trimester. Here's how:

The Symptoms

Double (or triple) the hormones can mean double the symptoms. Morning sickness that doesn't wait for morning. Exhaustion feels like someone unplugged your battery. Boobs are already preparing for a football team. And the bloating? You might be barely eight weeks and already feel like you've swallowed a whole watermelon. Don't be surprised if you start showing earlier. There's more going on in there, and your body wastes no time in adjusting.

The Monitoring

You'll likely be seen more often than someone carrying a singleton, and with good reason. Twin and multiple pregnancies come with different risks. Your team will want to keep a closer eye on growth, nutrition and how you're coping physically and emotionally. You may start to hear new terms like 'chorionicity' or 'monochorionic twins' – which basically means how many placentas and sacs are involved.

Don't worry, it will all be explained as you go, but it can feel like a lot at first.

The Reactions

Get ready for the unsolicited comments. 'Oh my God, double trouble!' 'You'll never sleep again!' 'Do twins run in your family?'

Everyone becomes very interested in your uterus. Some will mean well. Others will be dramatic. You're allowed to roll your eyes. You're allowed to be scared and excited. You're allowed to feel all the things – even if they all hit you before you've left the hospital car park.

The Planning

It's okay if your brain jumps straight to logistics. Do we need a new home? A double pram? Two cots? Should I start bulk-buying nappies now? The answer is: take it step by step. Not everything needs to be solved by week nine. Start small. Learn about the type of twin pregnancy you're having. Focus on nourishing yourself. Ask your midwife questions. And most importantly – rest. Not just physically, but emotionally. It's a lot to take in.

I'M PREGNANT ... NOW WHAT?

We talked earlier in the book about the rules around telling your employer you're pregnant, and those rules don't change if you are having twins, but it's worth noting that you may end up telling them a little earlier because you might show sooner and you will have more scans to attend. You don't have to say it's twins if you don't want to – you can simply explain that your team is keeping a closer eye on you and navigate it in whatever way feels right for you.

Pregnancy with multiples doesn't mean your joy is multiplied and your fear divided. Often, both joy *and* fear are doubled. That's normal. You've been given a lot to process and you're doing better than you think.

HYPEREMESIS GRAVIDARUM*

There's nausea in pregnancy, and then there's **Hyperemesis Gravidarum (HG)**. They are not the same thing. And I need to say that straight away. If you're reading this and going through it, I am *so sorry*. I don't even want to imagine how hard this chapter might be to read while you're in it. You are dealing with something that so many people don't understand unless they've lived it. You are not being dramatic. You are not exaggerating. And no, this is not 'just morning sickness'.

---

* This section discusses hyperemesis gravidarum and includes a real story that touches on pregnancy termination due to severe illness. Please read at your own pace and give yourself permission to pause or skip this section if you need to.

THE FIRST TRIMESTER

People love to talk about nausea like it's some pregnancy initiation. The jokes about ginger biscuits, the herbal tea suggestions, the classic 'have you tried dry toast before you get out of bed?' But HG doesn't care about your dry toast. It doesn't clock off at midday. It doesn't even give you a break between waves.

HG is another level. It's sickness so extreme it makes you question everything. Vomiting 20, 30, even 50 times a day. Not being able to keep down water. Ending up in hospital. Living off IV fluids. Losing weight. Losing energy. Losing your grip. It's when your body isn't just sick – it feels like it's turning against you.

And what makes it worse? People brush it off. Because nausea is 'normal', right? Because you don't *look* ill. Because unless someone sees you mid-vomit, it can be easy to pretend you're okay. And even then, they'll probably still smile and say, 'Ohhh morning sickness, eh?' No. Not morning sickness. Not even close. This is a diagnosis. A medical condition. A complete thief of joy, comfort and of the kind of pregnancy experience you might've hoped for. It's brutal. And it's real.

Women get admitted to hospital for this – some more than once. They're given anti-sickness meds that sometimes barely touch the sides. They're put on drips. Some need steroids. Some are so depleted they're kept hydrated through their veins because their stomach won't cooperate. Their skin is grey, their bodies exhausted – and their minds? Drained. Disconnected.

I'M PREGNANT ... NOW WHAT?

Some women choose to terminate their pregnancies because of it. Not because they don't want the baby, but because they physically, mentally and emotionally cannot cope with the suffering. And many women who go through it once decide never to get pregnant again. That's how deep the trauma can run.

HG increases the risk of postnatal depression. It affects bonding. It steals the glow people love to talk about. This is why I say – women with HG are some of the most *robbed* during pregnancy. If you're reading this and you're in the thick of it, please hear me when I say:

You're not weak.

You're not being negative.

You're surviving something that would bring most people to their knees. And you're still here.

If you're someone who isn't experiencing it, but you know someone who is, believe them. Please. Don't try to fix it with jokes or advice. Don't minimise it. Just be there. Just acknowledge what they're facing and hold space for it.

In some situations, pregnancy can become so overwhelming, so physically and emotionally draining, that it feels like an impossible choice between your own health and your baby's. It isn't something people talk about openly, but it is a reality for some women. Let me tell you about someone I know. A woman I love deeply. She wanted to share her story but asked to remain anonymous. She already had a little boy when she found out she was pregnant again. At first, she was happy. It wasn't planned, but she wasn't scared. Until

THE FIRST TRIMESTER

the sickness came. And when I say sickness, I'm talking about a kind of relentless, soul-draining, terrifying illness that stripped her down completely.

She told me: 'I thought I was going to die. I couldn't eat. I couldn't drink. I couldn't lift my head without vomiting. I couldn't care for my son. I couldn't care for myself. My body was shutting down.'

She kept trying. Kept hoping it would ease up. She did *everything* she could. But it didn't stop. And in the end, she said something I'll never forget: 'I felt like I had to choose. Me or the baby.'

She terminated the pregnancy.

Not because she didn't love. Not because she didn't care. But because she was being honest about what her body and mind could take. She had a child who needed her. And she needed herself.

She grieves that decision, because she felt helpless. She felt disregarded. Like no one was truly listening; like she had to make an impossible choice in a world that kept telling her it was just nausea.

And she wanted me to share this with you, exactly as she said it:

If you're reading this and you're in that place – I see you. I know how dark it can feel. I know how much you wish this was different. I had to make a decision I never thought I'd face. And I still carry it. But I also carried myself through something I didn't think I'd survive. You are not weak.

I'M PREGNANT ... NOW WHAT?

If you're in that space right now, whether you've got your head over a toilet or you're lying in bed afraid to move - please know I wrote this for you. This won't be the part people screenshot or share on Instagram. But it might be the one that makes someone feel *seen*. And if that's you - I hope you know that this is not your fault. That this isn't what you deserved. And that you don't owe anyone strength right now. Just hang on. Just survive. That's more than enough.

If you've made it through HG, whether you want to try again or never want to see a pregnancy test ever again, I see you too. Let this chapter stand as proof that you're not alone. You deserve softness. You deserve compassion. You deserve to rest. And you *never* deserve to hear the words, 'It's just morning sickness.'

SURROGACY OR GESTATIONAL CARRIER PREGNANCY – THE PERSPECTIVE SHIFT

Not every pregnancy is carried by the person who will raise the child. Some journeys involve surrogacy or gestational carriers, and while that might not apply to the majority of readers here, it absolutely deserves space in this book. For intended parents, there is often this strange in-between feeling - joy at expecting a baby but also a sense of distance because you are not the one physically carrying them. For the carrier, there is the daily reality of pregnancy, but with a different emotional backdrop, because this is not their baby to take home.

THE FIRST TRIMESTER

Surrogacy highlights just how many different ways families can be made and it shifts the perspective of pregnancy. It reminds us that the emotional and logistical side of pregnancy isn't one size fits all. There can be layers of gratitude, complexity and sometimes even grief. Grief for not being able to carry your own baby, or grief for the physical sacrifices made in carrying for someone else. Wherever you fall in that journey, you deserve acknowledgement, compassion and care.

If you are an intended parent who is not physically carrying the baby, it's completely normal to wonder how you'll bond. There are small but powerful ways to stay connected. You might attend scans and appointments where possible or ask for recordings of the heartbeat to keep with you. Some parents write letters or record voice notes to the baby during the pregnancy, so that when the time comes, the baby will already have a sense of their voice. Choosing items for the nursery or preparing special outfits can also make you feel more connected to the journey. And if you feel comfortable, gentle rituals with your surrogate - such as sharing updates or keeping a pregnancy journal together - can help you feel part of the experience.

These steps don't erase the complexity, but they can give you touchpoints of connection and control in a season that can sometimes feel out of your hands.

And if you are the surrogate, I want to use this moment to acknowledge your strength. Carrying a baby for someone else is a profound act of generosity and resilience. It is a gift that speaks to courage, compassion and the depth of what it means to support another family's dream.

PREGNANCY IN A LARGER OR OLDER BODY: FATPHOBIA AND AGEISM IN HEALTHCARE AND OWNING YOUR SPACE

At Mama's Classes (my antenatal classes and support network for mums), one of our guiding mottos is celebrating communities and individuals who are often overlooked in healthcare and in wider society. I would be doing myself a disservice if I did not include this section. Let me start by saying I have issues with Body Mass Index (BMI) charts. That is a rant for another day. But what I will say is that pregnancy in a bigger body can look and feel different, and unfortunately, the way healthcare professionals handle it is often clumsy, insensitive or downright unkind. There is a long way to go in how we talk to and care for women in larger bodies.

I have seen women made to feel ashamed in clinics and appointments. I have seen women downplay what they have eaten or outright lie, saying, 'Oh, I just had a tiny snack,' when really, they had a doughnut. Not because they are being difficult, but because they feel judged and unsafe in being honest. When that happens, healthcare has failed. Because if a woman feels too ashamed to speak the truth about her health, then we have closed the door to helping her properly.

Yes, there are things in pregnancy that can look different in bigger bodies. Scans can be more technically challenging.

THE FIRST TRIMESTER

Risks like gestational diabetes or blood pressure issues can be slightly higher. But how that information is delivered matters. You can give the same medical facts with dignity, kindness and partnership, or you can deliver them with shame and blame. Too often, women get the second option.

We are also seeing more women having babies later in life – over 35, sometimes over 40. The system slaps a label on it like 'geriatric pregnancy' or 'advanced maternal age' as if you are ancient because you are 36. Yes, care can look a little different in these pregnancies, with extra monitoring or extra scans, but again, how that is framed makes all the difference. It should never be about shaming or scaring – it should be about support.

So, what do you do if you feel that sting of discrimination in your care? My best advice is to stay honest, because hiding parts of your health history or choices only makes it harder for your team to support you properly. But honesty does not mean silence. You can be honest and still be assertive. If a comment makes you feel judged or dismissed, it is okay to say, 'I don't feel comfortable with how that was said,' or 'I'd like us to focus on the care I need, not my weight or my age.' You don't have to take on other people's projections as truth.

Bring someone with you to appointments if that helps you feel more supported. Write down your questions and your concerns ahead of time, so you don't get flustered in the moment. And remember, you are not 'difficult' for asking to be treated with respect.

Pregnancy is already a vulnerable journey. No woman should ever feel like she has failed before she has even started, just because of her age or her body size. I can't change the healthcare system overnight, but you deserve care that is safe, kind and respectful.

PREGNANCY AFTER FERTILITY TREATMENTS – ADJUSTING TO 'NORMAL' AFTER A MEDICALISED JOURNEY

Pregnancy after fertility treatments, such as IVF, comes with its own set of emotions. For many women, the journey to get here was long, medicalised and exhausting. Endless blood tests, injections, scans, appointments, waiting and hoping. Then finally, that positive test. But here's the thing – it can be hard to suddenly switch from a world where everything was controlled, measured and medical, into what feels like a 'normal' pregnancy.

I've seen so many women who feel like they've still got 'IVF pregnancy' stamped across their foreheads. It is almost like you carry that label the whole way through, even though once you are pregnant, many IVF pregnancies are just as straightforward as any other. Sometimes the medical side was just the help you needed to get pregnant in the first place, and now the pregnancy itself can unfold beautifully on its own.

But that adjustment takes time. There can be an extra layer of anxiety, especially if the road to get here involved years of trying or loss. It is natural to find yourself over-thinking every twinge, every scan result, every symptom. That's not you being paranoid – it's you coming down from years of having every step monitored under a microscope.

Here is what I want to encourage you to do: enjoy the pregnancy. Celebrate it. Allow yourself to soak up the moments without always waiting for something to go wrong. You're pregnant – full stop. That's worth holding on to.

Please, don't fall into the trap of thinking you now have to overcompensate to prove you're a great mum. I've noticed that a lot of mums who have been through IVF or other treatments put so much pressure on themselves afterwards. They're the ones brands love, because they know these mums often want that little extra reassurance, that little extra something to say, 'You're doing it right.' But you don't need to buy anything or perform in any way to prove your worth.

Your journey here might have been full of medicine, science and procedures, but your pregnancy and birth don't have to be. You can still have a calm, beautiful, non-medicalised experience. And whether it looks picture-perfect or a little messy, it's still yours. IVF might be part of your story, but it does not define your pregnancy.

WRAPPING UP THE MADNESS THAT IS TRIMESTER ONE

And breathe.

If you've made it this far through the first trimester, I hope you're feeling a little more informed, a little more reassured and a lot more seen. Because listen, this part of pregnancy? It's a whirlwind. Your body's working overtime, your mind is trying to catch up, and your emotions are doing gymnastics.

You've probably googled a thousand things. You've maybe panicked over a cramp, cried over an advert or wondered if eating that soft cheese five weeks ago has doomed everything. Maybe you've already bought a pram. Or maybe you've just been trying to keep toast down. No matter how it's been for you, you're doing just fine.

This chapter wasn't meant to fix everything or take away every single fear. But I hope it helped you say, 'Okay, I get what's happening now.' I hope you've laughed at least once. I hope you've felt held. And I really hope you know you're not alone.

There's so much more to come, but for now, whether you're bloated, glowing, exhausted or thriving (or all four at once), I want you to know: You are doing something extraordinary.

So, grab a snack, go easy on yourself, and I'll see you in the second trimester – where the symptoms might ease up a bit, the bump might start to show, and yes ... the chaos continues.

PART 2

THE SECOND TRIMESTER

HELLO BUMP!

Welcome to the second trimester, arguably the fastest-moving part of pregnancy. One minute you're telling people your news, and the next you're wondering how you're already halfway there. This is what many people call the *'high' of pregnancy* – your bump is making its debut, the early nausea (hopefully) has eased up, and you might even have that famous 'glow' people talk about.

It's a time when a lot of women say they *actually* enjoy being pregnant – your energy's back (or at least better than before), you're starting to feel those first little flutters, and you can eat without needing a bucket nearby. In this chapter, we're going to chat about everything from the scans you might be offered, to the so-called baby glow, to planning a babymoon if you fancy one, plus a bunch of other bits you might not have thought about but will absolutely want to know.

I'M PREGNANT ... NOW WHAT?

PHYSICAL CHANGES IN THE SECOND TRIMESTER

All right, let's talk about the physical stuff – the changes you can *see* and *feel*. The second trimester is when things really start to take shape ... literally. If this is your first baby, you might have only just started noticing a little curve in your belly towards the end of the first trimester, but now? The bump is here to make its presence known. If it's your second (or third or more), you might have spotted it earlier, but this is still the phase where it starts to properly pop and say, 'Yep, we're doing this.'

At the start of this trimester, you might notice something funny – some days it feels like you have no bump at all, and other days you're suddenly asking yourself, 'Where did this bump come from?' A lot of that can depend on things like what you've eaten, how much you've bloated, or even just how your baby's positioned that day. It's a bit of an up-and-down, surprise-each-morning situation.

Clothes start fitting differently, and this is the point where you might actually find yourself undoing the button of your jeans after lunch. Your body is stretching, shifting and making space for the growing human inside you. Your breasts are joining in too – filling out your bra, feeling heavier and gearing up for their feeding role later on.

This is also the time the 'pregnancy nose' can make her debut, where your nose may look a little puffier or wider, thanks to hormonal changes and increased blood flow. Yes, even your nose wants to get involved in the pregnancy. It's just another one of those random, slightly surprising changes that can pop up during pregnancy. This is the trimester where pregnancy may stop being a secret.

SKIN CHANGES: HYPERPIGMENTATION, STRETCH MARKS AND THE 'GLOW'

Let's talk skin. The second trimester is when you might start noticing a few changes – some you'll love, some you might side-eye in the mirror.

Hyperpigmentation – This happens because pregnancy hormones like oestrogen and progesterone increase melanin production, the pigment that gives skin its colour. Areas that naturally have more pigment, like your face, armpits, inner thighs or the line down your belly (linea nigra), might darken even more. If you're a skincare babe, now's the time to stick to gentle products, no harsh experiments here.

The 'Pregnancy Glow' – For some women, it's real. Skin looks plump, dewy and hydrated. That's because those same hormones make your oil glands more active, giving your skin that sheen. For others, that extra oil production can mean clogged pores and breakouts instead. It's basically your body flipping a hormonal coin.

Stretch marks – They appear when your skin's middle layer stretches faster than it can keep up with, causing tiny tears that show up as streaks. Genetics play a big role – if your skin type is more prone, no cream in the world can stop them completely. Staying moisturised can help your skin feel comfortable and reduce itchiness, but if you get stretch marks, you get stretch marks. It's such a shame that society has made us think a natural, powerful change is somehow 'ugly'. Your body is doing something incredible, and you're beautiful with your stretch marks – full stop.

CHANGES IN APPETITE AND WEIGHT GAIN: NAVIGATING HUNGER, CRAVINGS AND FOOD GUILT

One of the reasons people say they *love* the second trimester is because, for many, the morning sickness (or 'all-day sickness') finally eases up. Your appetite comes back, food starts tasting good again and you can actually enjoy a meal without side-eyeing the nearest bin. It's like you've been reunited with your taste buds.

This is often the stage where cravings kick in properly – not just 'I fancy something sweet' but 'I need this exact brand of chocolate bar *right now or I can't sleep.*' Some people find themselves loving foods they used to hate, while others suddenly can't stand things they used to eat daily. It's all down to the hormonal shifts and your body's way of nudging you towards certain nutrients.

THE SECOND TRIMESTER

Naturally, with a better appetite comes weight gain – something that's completely normal and healthy at this stage. But I know a lot of women feel pressure or guilt around it, especially in a world where everyone has an opinion about bodies. Here's the truth: your body is working overtime, creating a tiny human inside you, your blood volume is increasing, your uterus is expanding and you've got extra fluid on board. Weight gain isn't just 'fat' – it's the literal building blocks your baby needs to grow.

If you find yourself feeling guilty after eating, remind yourself that food is fuel, *especially* now. Pregnancy is not the time for crash diets or food restriction. It's about balance, listening to your body's hunger cues, enjoying your cravings in moderation and knowing that it's okay if you go through phases of eating the same meal every single day.

FEELING THE BABY MOVE – WHAT THOSE FIRST FLUTTERS ACTUALLY FEEL LIKE

This is the trimester where you might start feeling those first little flutters – your baby's debut performance. At first, it's not the dramatic kick people imagine. It's more like bubbles popping, gentle taps or a goldfish flicking around inside you. Sometimes you feel them, sometimes you don't – not because your baby's not moving, but because they're still so tiny that their movements aren't always strong enough for you to notice.

For some women, these first kicks are pure magic – they can't get enough of them. For others, the feeling is weird.

And that's okay. Every time we run my antenatal classes, one of the icebreakers is asking what people love most about pregnancy and what they can't wait to be done with. Kicks almost always make it onto the 'love' list, though, for a few, they sneak onto the 'not a fan' side instead.

At this stage, there's no predictable rhythm to your baby's movements – they're still finding their groove. For most people, regular, more consistent movements become noticeable from around 24 weeks onwards.

That's when you'll start picking up on your baby's patterns and be able to recognise their 'usual' activity. Until then, enjoy (or at least observe) these early, unpredictable little hellos from inside.

BACKACHE AND POSTURE SHIFTS: WHY YOUR BACK HATES YOU AND HOW TO SHOW IT LOVE

By the second trimester, your body's centre of gravity has officially shifted – and your back knows it. Your bump is growing week by week, your spine is working overtime to adjust to the new weight at the front and the pregnancy hormone relaxin is quietly loosening your ligaments and joints in preparation for birth. On paper, it's very clever biology – your body is literally making itself more flexible so your pelvis can open up when the time comes. In reality, it can also make you feel wobbly, unstable and achy, like your lower back is considering sending you a formal letter of complaint.

THE SECOND TRIMESTER

It's important to know the difference between a general pregnancy backache and something more specific called **Symphysis Pubis Dysfunction** (SPD), also known as Pelvic Girdle Pain (see page 135). A standard pregnancy backache is usually a dull, persistent ache across your lower back, the kind that gets worse after you've been standing for a long time, sitting awkwardly or trying to carry the weekly shop. SPD, on the other hand, is in a league of its own. It tends to feel sharper and more targeted, often starting in the very front or centre of your pelvis and sometimes radiating into your hips, inner thighs or even down to your knees. It can make walking, climbing stairs or even rolling over in bed a painful mission.

SPD happens because the pelvic joints become too loose – thanks to all that lovely relaxin – and start moving unevenly, putting strain on the surrounding muscles and ligaments. It's not something you should 'push through' or just accept as part of pregnancy. If you're struggling, speak to your midwife or GP and ask for a referral to a physiotherapist. Physiotherapy can make a huge difference – teaching you exercises to strengthen the right muscles, showing you how to move in ways that reduce strain, and giving you tips to avoid triggering pain in the first place. If you can afford it, seeing a private physio means you can often get help faster and more regularly.

In the meantime, there are plenty of ways to show your back some love. Pregnancy-safe massage can help release tension, improve circulation and simply make you feel human again (even if it's just a partner giving you a gentle lower back rub with some oil). Being mindful of your posture – avoiding standing with your belly pushed forward like you're posing for a maternity shoot and steering clear of slumping into the sofa for hours – can also help more than you think. A maternity support belt can provide extra stability by taking some of the weight off your pelvis and lower back. Gentle, low-impact activities like swimming, prenatal yoga or short, slow walks will keep your muscles engaged without overloading your already hard-working joints.

The bottom line? Your back is carrying a heavier load than it's ever had to before. Treat it with kindness now, and it's far more likely to forgive you later.

NASAL CONGESTION

I honestly thought I could skip nasal congestion when I was planning out this chapter, but why did I even think that? It's so common in the second trimester that it deserves its own spotlight. (And you thought 'pregnancy nose' was the only time your nose would take centre stage!)

Many women find themselves feeling constantly bunged up, like they've got a lingering cold that never quite goes away. This happens because during pregnancy the tissue inside your nose swells. Increased blood flow and hormone changes – particularly oestrogen – make the tiny blood vessels in your nasal passages expand. That swelling narrows the airways, which makes you feel congested. Some people even lose part of their sense of smell or notice their voice sounds different – like they've suddenly caught a cold that refuses to leave.

With more blood flowing through your body (remember, you've got almost 50 per cent more blood volume in pregnancy), your nasal vessels are more fragile too, which is why nosebleeds are so much more common. For some women, it's just the occasional one when they blow their nose. For others, it feels like their nose has suddenly turned into a leaky tap.

The frustrating part is that not every over-the-counter remedy is safe in pregnancy, so you can't just grab your usual decongestants. That's why nasal congestion can feel so stressful – you're uncomfortable, you might be snoring (which your partner will definitely notice), and the relief options are limited. But here's the science-y bit that actually helps:

- Staying hydrated thins mucus and makes it easier to clear.
- Using a humidifier or steaming can keep your nasal passages moist.
- Saline sprays are safe and can help rinse things out.
- Sleeping slightly propped up can make breathing easier at night.

While it's annoying, it usually eases up after birth. Until then, keep tissues on standby and maybe warn your partner about the extra snoring.

MEDICAL AND HEALTH TOPICS

THE ANOMALY SCAN
(AKA THE 20-WEEK SCAN)

Let's start with one of the biggest medical moments of the second trimester: the anomaly scan, also called the 20-week scan. This is a detailed ultrasound where the sonographer takes their time checking over your baby from head to tiny little toes. They're not just looking to confirm your baby's sex or show you a cute profile picture for your fridge; they're carefully examining your baby's organs, bones and facial features to make sure everything is developing as it should. They'll measure different parts of the baby's body, check the position of the placenta, and look at the amniotic fluid levels too.

At around 20 weeks, your baby is developed enough for their organs, bones and major structures to be clearly visible on the scan, but still small enough that the sonographer can get a good look at everything without your baby being too big and curled up. It's that sweet spot within your pregnancy journey where detail meets visibility, making it the ideal time to pick up on any potential issues.

The purpose is to detect any structural conditions or abnormalities early on. For most people, everything is fine and it's simply a reassuring moment to see your baby in such detail. But if something unexpected is spotted, this scan can shape what happens next. Results from this scan may mean you're offered additional scans, more frequent monitoring or referrals to specialists so your pregnancy can be supported in the best way possible.

In many low-risk pregnancies, this is actually the *last* scan you'll be offered on the NHS. If everything looks healthy, you may not have another routine ultrasound unless a concern pops up later in the pregnancy. That's why this appointment feels like such a milestone – it's both a detailed medical check-up and, for a lot of parents, the last time they'll 'see' their baby before the big day.

CERCLAGE: WHEN A STITCH HOLDS MORE THAN JUST THE CERVIX

For some women, the second trimester brings up something called a cerclage, also known as a cervical stitch. It's a procedure where doctors put a stitch around the cervix to help keep it closed, usually because it's been found to be short, weak or already starting to thin too early. The goal is simple: to help prevent a premature birth or late miscarriage.

There are a few different scenarios where a cerclage might be offered. Sometimes it's for mums who've never had a miscarriage before, but a routine scan shows their cervix is shorter than expected and at risk of opening early (a condition known as cervical weakness). Other times, it's offered to women who, sadly, have had pregnancy losses in the past, where cervical weakness may have been a contributing factor. In those cases, the stitch is both a preventative measure and a reassurance.

Having a cerclage can completely change the trajectory of a pregnancy. A lot of women are advised to rest more, sometimes even to the point of strict bed rest, depending on how their cervix is holding up, and that can be really tough physically, emotionally and mentally. It can take away that freedom to enjoy pregnancy the way you imagined.

I think about mums who are so excited to share their pregnancy online, planning to post every milestone, every bump picture, every joyful update. But once they find out their cervix is thinning and a stitch is placed, their whole experience changes. Instead of joy, it becomes fear. Every day is a question: Is my cervix going to open? Will my baby come too soon? Especially for women who've experienced loss before, that constant uncertainty can feel like pregnancy has been stolen from them.

A cerclage doesn't erase fear, but it does give the cervix a stronger chance of holding on until baby is viable and stronger. For many women, it works well and helps them reach a much safer stage in pregnancy. But it's okay to acknowledge the emotional weight of living with it – and the way it can feel like you're holding your breath for weeks on end. If you're someone who's offered a cerclage, know this: you're not alone. It's not your fault. Even though your pregnancy might look different from how you imagined, the stitch is there to give your baby the best possible chance.

THE SECOND TRIMESTER

MID-PREGNANCY BLOODS AND URINE TESTS

By the second trimester, the routine of antenatal appointments is in full swing, and there's one thing you can bet on at almost every visit: we're going to check your blood pressure, and we're going to ask you for a urine sample. Every. Single. Time. It might feel repetitive, but these quick checks can pick up on conditions like pre-eclampsia, which can sometimes develop with little to no symptoms in the early stages. The first sign might be a rise in your blood pressure or the presence of protein in your urine.

TOP TIP

Make life easier for yourself and be prepared. I know a lot of mums say, 'But I've already peed before my appointment!' which is why I always recommend this little trick. At your appointment, ask for an extra urine sample cup to take home. Keep it clean and ready. On the morning of your *next* appointment, don't pee first thing. Instead, pee in the cup before you leave the house (make sure to seal it tightly afterwards to avoid leaks!), bring it with you and hand it in when you arrive. That way, you're not sitting in the waiting room sipping water and praying your bladder cooperates.

Blood tests also pop up in the second trimester, though not as often as in the first. These might include checking your iron levels, screening for gestational diabetes if you're at risk or following up on anything that came back borderline earlier in your pregnancy. These routine check-ups might feel small, but they're one of the most powerful tools we have to make sure both you and your baby are staying healthy as your pregnancy progresses.

GESTATIONAL DIABETES SCREENING: WHO GETS TESTED AND WHY

Gestational diabetes (GDM) is a type of diabetes that only happens in pregnancy. It means your blood sugar levels are higher than they should be, and it happens because pregnancy hormones can make it harder for your body to use insulin properly. Insulin is the hormone that helps control your blood sugar, and when your body can't use it effectively, your sugar levels rise.

Some people are automatically offered a gestational diabetes test because their risk is higher. This includes anyone who is Black, South Asian or from certain other ethnic backgrounds, anyone who is considered obese, those with a family history of diabetes, anyone who's had gestational diabetes in a previous pregnancy or those who've previously had a large baby. GDM can affect *anyone*, however. I've seen slim, white women with no family history get diagnosed, so you can't assume you're 'safe' just because you don't fit the so-called risk profile.

THE SECOND TRIMESTER

There are usually two main tests: one is a random blood sugar check, and the other, which is the more common, is the **oral glucose tolerance test (OGTT)**. The OGTT is the one most people talk about because it involves 'the drink'. For some women, it's genuinely fine. Sweet but drinkable, especially if it's been chilled. For others, it's like liquid jelly gone wrong, and they'll tell you it's horrendous. It really depends on your taste buds and, honestly, on your hospital. Different places use slightly different drinks.

OGTT: WHAT TO EXPECT

Here's how the OGTT usually works: you'll be asked to fast from the night before, meaning no food and no sugary drinks (water is fine). When you arrive, they'll take a blood sample to see your fasting blood sugar level. Then you'll be given the glucose drink – usually about the sweetness of a very syrupy squash – to down within a set amount of time. After that, you'll wait, normally for two hours, without eating or drinking anything else. Then they'll take another blood sample to see how your body has processed the sugar. If your levels are higher than the healthy range, you'll be diagnosed with gestational diabetes.

I'M PREGNANT ... NOW WHAT?

I know from speaking to so many pregnant women that this diagnosis can feel like the end of the world. But it's not. For a lot of women, gestational diabetes can be managed with dietary changes such as reducing refined sugar, spacing out carbs through the day, and balancing meals with protein and fibre. This isn't about 'you failed' or 'you ate badly' - it's hormones. Your placenta produces hormones that make your body less sensitive to insulin, and for some women, that's enough to tip the balance, no matter how healthy they eat. I've had women tell me they ate one slice of bread and their sugar spiked as if they'd had four doughnuts and a can of full-fat Coke. That's how much your body can struggle with it. It's not a reflection of your effort, discipline or worth.

Some women will need medication or insulin if diet alone doesn't keep their sugar levels where they need to be. The goal is to keep your blood sugar in a safe range for both you and your baby, and your midwife or diabetes team will guide you through it. If you do get diagnosed, you'll usually be offered extra scans and closer monitoring to make sure your baby is growing at a healthy rate.

The bottom line is that gestational diabetes is common but manageable, and it doesn't make you a bad mother or mean your pregnancy is doomed. It just means your body needs a bit of extra support to keep both you and your baby healthy.

THE SECOND TRIMESTER

VACCINATIONS DURING PREGNANCY: FLU JAB, WHOOPING COUGH AND WHY THEY MATTER

I get asked about vaccines in pregnancy *a lot*. And here's the funny thing: 90 per cent of the people who ask already know what they're going to do. My role isn't to tell you what decision to make – it's to give you the facts about what these vaccines are, what they're aimed at and why they're offered so you can make an informed choice.

The two main ones are:

- **The flu jab** – offered during flu season to protect you from catching flu, which can be more serious in pregnancy and increase the risk of complications for you and your baby.
- **The whooping cough (pertussis) vaccine** – usually offered between 16 and 32 weeks. This helps your body produce antibodies that cross the placenta to your baby, giving them protection in those first few months before they're old enough for their own vaccines.

I have to address the conspiracy theories, because I've heard them all, even the 'these vaccines are actually trackers' one. I would be *so* annoyed if the NHS were putting trackers in vaccines while still struggling to fix the computer in the antenatal clinic that's been broken for seven months.

Or if they had the budget for microchips while the revolving door with the 'use other door' sign has been broken for three years. Let's be real – if they can't fix that, they're probably not running a nationwide spy system through your arm.

One thing I *am* against, though, is the constant pushing and nagging I've seen in some clinics, especially with the whooping cough vaccine. I've met midwives who badger women so much you'd think they were getting paid on commission. That's not okay. I do genuinely believe these vaccines are important, but I also believe you should *never* be forced into something you don't want. The best decision is one you've made because you understand it, not because someone wore you down. In the end, these vaccines are offered to protect you and your baby at a time when your immune system is naturally working differently. Whether you say yes or no is your choice, but if you do take them, it's because you've decided it's right for you, not because someone in a uniform wouldn't take 'no' for an answer.

SEX DURING PREGNANCY: MYTHS, SAFETY AND SHIFTING LIBIDO

The second trimester is often called the 'sweet spot' of pregnancy, and for some women, that definitely applies to their sex life. Pregnancy hormones can increase blood flow to your pelvic area, making you feel more sensitive and, for some, more interested in sex than they have in months. Your libido might be higher, your body might feel more

THE SECOND TRIMESTER

responsive and you might find you're enjoying intimacy in a different way. Of course, not everyone feels this, and that's completely normal too. Libido in pregnancy is personal, and it can change from week to week.

Let's deal with one of the most common questions I get: is it safe? For most women with uncomplicated pregnancies, yes, sex is completely safe. Your baby is well protected inside the amniotic sac and the muscles of the uterus. Before you're even going to ask, let me put this one to rest: no matter how endowed your partner is, he's not poking that baby, okay? Unless he can bend, shift, and somehow find his way through to that (in which case *he's* the one who'll need to go to Accident and Emergency), it's just not happening.

There are some cases where your midwife or doctor might recommend avoiding sex, such as if you have placenta praevia, unexplained bleeding or a risk of pre-term labour. Otherwise, it's safe, and any changes in your comfort level are more likely down to position, bump size or just how you're feeling that day.

Remember – intimacy doesn't always have to mean sex. For some couples, especially in pregnancy, intimacy might look like massages, long hugs, back rubs, lying next to each other watching a film or simply enjoying each other's company. It's about connection, not just the physical act, so find what works for both of you right now. The bottom line? Your body will tell you what it's up for. If your libido's high, enjoy it. If it's low, that's fine too. And if you and your partner are willing to get creative with positions or redefine what intimacy looks like, the second trimester can be a pretty fun time.

COMMON SECOND TRIMESTER COMPLICATIONS

I'm not here to worry you, and I'm definitely not about to dump every worst-case scenario on your head, but I also believe that knowledge is power. There are certain conditions that can pop up in the second trimester where you or your baby might just need a little more support.

One of those is something called *placenta praevia*, where the placenta is sitting low in the womb and covering the cervix (the exit, basically). For a lot of mummies, this sorts itself out as the uterus grows and the placenta shifts upwards, but if it doesn't, especially if it's *completely* covering the cervix, it can block the baby's way out, which makes vaginal birth unsafe and changes the type of care you'll receive. You might be offered a planned C-section, and your team will keep a closer eye on you, especially in the later stages.

Another example is an *incompetent cervix* (which, by the way, is a rude name if you ask me), where the cervix starts shortening or opening too early. It can increase

> the risk of premature labour, but if it's spotted, there are options like vaginal progesterone or a cervical stitch to support the pregnancy and reduce that risk. Again, this isn't about causing fear. It's about knowing what might come up, so if it ever *does*, you're not blindsided.

DENTAL CARE DURING PREGNANCY: WHY GUMS MIGHT BLEED AND TEETH MIGHT ACHE

Listen, let me say this right now: one of the most important things you need to know, especially here in the UK, is that you're entitled to *free* NHS dental care during your pregnancy. Yes, *free*. Now, am I guaranteeing you'll get a dentist appointment right away? Nope, there could absolutely be a waiting list or difficulty booking. But in theory, the care is free, and you *can* push for it when you need it. Now, you won't get implants, crowns or whitening done for free, but what *is* available are check-ups, fillings, extractions and basic restorative work as needed to keep things manageable. It's about prevention, not glam upgrades.

There is no pain quite like dental pain. It's a *special* kind of agony. I've had women tell me it's worse than labour, and honestly, I believe them. I've felt it – the kind that makes you question every life choice up to that point. I've even promised (in a not-so-calm moment) that my future children would never, ever eat sweets. There was this one stubborn tooth so bad that I thought, *There's no way this tooth is going to heaven. If teeth were judged, it's going straight to hell.* Absolutely chaotic.

All the more reason to get your teeth checked during the second trimester – now, *before* it becomes a crisis. During pregnancy, your gums are more likely to bleed (thanks to those ramped-up pregnancy hormones and increased blood flow), and your teeth might feel extra sensitive even on a gentle day. Pain relief options during pregnancy are more limited than usual too, so dealing with a dental issue later? It's not just painful, it's a headache. Literally.

THE EMOTIONAL 'MIDDLE GROUND': NOT NEW TO PREGNANCY, NOT NEAR THE END EITHER

The second trimester is what I like to call the emotional middle ground. You're not new to pregnancy any more, but you're not close to the end either. It's that in-between stage where you can't quite see the finish line, but you've also left the starting point behind. It's a bit like being on a long-haul flight. Take-off is done, landing is ages away, and you're just ... cruising. You might look around and think, *So, what am I supposed to do now?* That's when the thoughts start creeping in – *What should I be doing? What haven't I done yet? Am I nearly there? Should I be panicking?*

Honestly, I think this is the time to slow down and just enjoy the bliss of pregnancy while it's not so heavy with symptoms.

THE SECOND TRIMESTER

In today's world, most of the things you suddenly realise you 'need' can be ordered with next-day delivery. There's no need to let the to-do list eat up your peace. Use this stage to breathe, relax and enjoy where you are right now.

BONDING WITH BABY: WHAT'S REAL AND WHAT'S FLUFF

It's never too early to start bonding with your baby. By the second trimester, your baby's ears are developing enough to start picking up sounds from the outside world – your voice, your partner's voice, music, even the rhythm of your heartbeat. They're not sitting in there thinking, *Wow, Mum's got great taste in Afrobeats*, but they are becoming familiar with the tones and patterns they hear most often.

Talking to your baby, singing to them and playing music you love can all be part of that bonding process. And rubbing your belly? That's not just fluff. Physical touch releases feel-good hormones like oxytocin, which help you feel connected to your baby and can even have a calming effect on you both.

For many mums, bonding feels easier at this stage because the bump is visible and those first flutters are starting – there's something to *see* and *feel*. It's a tangible reminder that there's a little person growing inside you, which makes talking or singing to them feel more natural. Whether it's a goodnight chat, a favourite playlist or just absentmindedly rubbing your bump while you watch TV, these small moments help you start building a relationship with your baby before they're even here.

CHOOSING ANTENATAL CLASSES: WHAT TO LOOK FOR AND WHEN TO BOOK

Let's start with antenatal classes. Now, if for some strange, crazy, unfathomable reason you don't want to go with Mama's Classes – whether that's one of our in-person sessions here in the UK or my online course (which, by the way, is amazing) – and you decide to go elsewhere, that's fine. At the end of the day, it's the same space: you're reading the book, you're getting the information and I'd much rather you learn from someone than not learn at all. But if you *are* shopping around for classes, there are a few things worth looking out for.

The most important thing? **Who's teaching it.** Please, please make sure you know who's standing at the front of the room giving you advice. Is it a qualified midwife or someone with proper training and experience, or just a 'birth coach' with no regulated background? It matters. Because I've heard horrendous stories from women about the things they were told in mainstream antenatal classes – things that are not only unhelpful, but in some cases, completely inaccurate. When you're pregnant, the last thing you need is wild, misleading information being dressed up as fact. So do your homework: speak to other mums who've

THE SECOND TRIMESTER

actually attended, check reviews and don't be afraid to ask questions before you book. The person running the class should be transparent about their qualifications and what their course covers.

Then think about **the content**. A solid antenatal class should prepare you for labour, birth and those first weeks with your baby. That means pain relief, feeding, partner roles, recovery and real-life tips – not just breathing exercises and relaxation.

Timing matters too. Most women book their classes to fall somewhere between 28 and 34 weeks, so the info is fresh in your mind but not so close to your due date that baby might beat you to it. Leave it too late, and you risk missing out.

Finally, consider **the vibe**. Some classes are very formal, some are relaxed and chatty, and some focus on helping you make friends with other parents-to-be. Choose the one that feels like your space.

Bottom line: antenatal classes should empower you with knowledge, not confuse you with nonsense. Whether you come to me (the best option, let's be honest) or go elsewhere, make sure you're learning from someone who knows what they're talking about.

TRAVELLING WHILE PREGNANT: FLIGHTS, LONG DRIVES AND INSURANCE CONSIDERATIONS

Let's talk about travelling in pregnancy, because this is one of the things I get messaged about constantly. Honestly, if

I'M PREGNANT ... NOW WHAT?

I could make money off the number of women who have panic-messaged me about flights, I'd be retired by now. I've had people crying at the airport, being turned away, and one lady in particular still sticks in my mind. She went to the airport in her crop top, bump out, ready for her holiday, thinking, *I'm in my second trimester, I'm fine.* But here's the truth: if you don't have a 'fit-to-fly' form, airlines can refuse to let you board. It doesn't matter how many weeks pregnant you are. Without that letter from your midwife or doctor, some airlines simply won't take the risk.

So please – if you know you're going to fly, make sure you organise a fit-to-fly form well in advance. Different airlines have different rules, and while most allow you to travel without question until around 28 weeks, many can still ask for proof earlier. Save yourself the tears at check-in.

Now, if you're thinking about a babymoon (just a fancy word for a holiday before the baby arrives), I'm a big believer that the second trimester is the perfect time to go. You've got enough of a bump to prove you're on a babymoon (and to get those extra smiles at the hotel), but you're not yet weighed down by the tiredness, heaviness and aches that often hit in the third trimester. Leave it too late, and you'll regret trying to waddle through airport security with swollen ankles. Travel in pregnancy can be done and can even be enjoyable – just make sure you've got the right paperwork, the right timing and you're looking after yourself on the journey.

Of course, it's not just about flights. Long drives can also take a toll, so make sure you're stopping regularly to stretch, walk and keep your circulation moving. Don't forget to check that your travel insurance actually covers pregnancy-related issues, because some policies sneakily don't.

Whether you're flying or stuck in the car, pregnancy increases your risk of blood clots (deep vein thrombosis or DVT). That's because your blood naturally becomes more 'sticky' in pregnancy as a way to protect you from bleeding too much during birth. Clever design, but the downside is it raises your risk of clots if you sit still for too long. That's why it's so important to stand up, stretch and move around regularly on long journeys. Think of it as medicine disguised as a leg stretch – you're literally keeping your blood flowing and lowering your risk. Compression socks can help, too. They're not the most glamorous or the most comfortable, but they're effective at improving circulation and reducing swelling, giving your body an extra nudge to keep blood moving when you're sitting still.

CREATING A BABY REGISTRY: ESSENTIALS VS. AESTHETIC DISTRACTIONS

This is the stage when, honestly, *shit's getting real*. In the first trimester, I told you not to worry about buying things just yet, but now's a good time to start thinking about what you actually want and need. And let me just say, I'm a big believer in registries. People are going to ask you, 'What do you need? What can I get you?' so make it easy for them. Share your registry, send it out if you want to. There's no shame in letting people buy you things that will actually help you.

Now, when it comes to what goes on the registry, it really depends on you. I'll be honest: I want a very pretty pram. A *beautiful* pram. That's just me – it makes me happy. But whether something ends up on your registry or you are buying it yourself, it's not about what's trendy or what looks fancy; it's about what works for you. Think about what is practical, what fits your space and what genuinely brings you joy.

So when you're building your registry, think about the essentials you'll definitely use, but don't be afraid to add things that make you smile, too. Essentials are practical, aesthetics are personal – but neither defines your worth as a parent.

If something isn't within your budget, don't stretch yourself to get it. Your baby doesn't *need* an expensive pram, cot or changing table to be loved and cared for. Whether your baby is pushed around in a beige designer pram or a sturdy, no-frills one, you're still a good mum.

What really matters is that it's safe, it works for your lifestyle and fits your budget. And if you're on a tight budget, please don't feel bad about buying second-hand, or accepting hand-me-downs or pre-loved bits. Babies grow quickly, and so many baby items barely get used before they are passed on. There is no shame in choosing what works for you and your reality.

BABY NAME TALKS – HOW TO HAVE THEM WITHOUT FULL-BLOWN ARGUMENTS

So, let's say, for some strange reason, you're having a baby girl and you *don't* want to name her Elizabeth after a certain famous midwife (I mean, questionable choice, but fine). Then yes, it's time to start talking about baby names. And honestly, I think this is one of the nicer, lighter parts of pregnancy. It doesn't all have to be symptoms and scans – this is a chance to get a bit cute and playful with what you'd love to call your baby.

I've seen baby name talks turn into full-blown arguments. One person's 'perfect' name is the other person's 'absolutely not'. So, my advice? Treat it like a fun conversation, not a battle. Write down your lists, share your ideas, laugh at the ridiculous ones and remember you're both on the same team.

Different cultures approach naming very differently. I once went to a naming ceremony where – I kid you not – that baby had about 20 names. Each one had meaning, history and family importance. It reminded me that naming isn't just about style – it can also be about identity, heritage and honouring your people. So whether your baby ends up with one carefully chosen name or a whole line-up of them, keep the process joyful.

UNIQUE JOURNEYS FOR THE SECOND TRIMESTER

In this section, we'll explore some of the unique journeys that can shape the second trimester. From preparing older siblings for the arrival of a new baby to navigating the mix of guilt and excitement that pregnancy can bring. Each of these experiences is valid, and each brings its own set of feelings and decisions.

My hope is that wherever you find yourself – whether this is your first baby, your fifth or a long-awaited pregnancy after loss or treatment – you see yourself reflected in these pages. The second trimester is not just about a growing bump, it is about growing into this new journey in all its forms.

PREPARING OLDER SIBLINGS: GUILT, EXCITEMENT AND TODDLER LOGIC

If this isn't your first baby, then pregnancy comes with a whole extra layer: preparing older siblings. And toddlers? Whew. Toddlers will humble you. One minute they're hugging your bump saying, 'Baby in Mummy's tummy,' the next they're announcing your news to strangers in Tesco

THE SECOND TRIMESTER

because toddlers genuinely thrive on telling people things they did *not* need to know. If you've been trying to keep the pregnancy quiet, good luck. Toddlers are not bound by NDAs.

Honestly, I don't know what it is, but I feel like second-borns come out like soldiers. They've had to put up with a lot from the womb – dodging toddler elbows, bouncy cuddles and endless pokes at your bump. Teaching toddlers how to be gentle with the bump is its own mission, because they just don't have a sense of danger. What feels like a 'soft' pat to them can feel like a wrestling move to you. So it's about modelling gentleness, showing them how to stroke your tummy lightly, and reminding them over and over (and over) again.

There can also be a bit of guilt in this stage. You might find yourself worrying about how your older child will cope with sharing your attention, or if they'll feel left out when the baby arrives. That's normal. At the same time, there's often a lot of excitement too – children can surprise you with how loving and protective they become, even at a young age. The trick is to make it fun and simple: let them pat your tummy gently while saying 'baby', show them pictures of babies or read storybooks about becoming a big brother or sister. Give them little 'jobs' so they feel included – helping choose a babygrow, singing to the bump or practising with a doll.

And through it all, reassure them that there will always be space for them. Because underneath the chaos of toddler logic, what they really want to know is that they're still loved and just as important, even with a new baby coming.

> ## WELCOMING BABY: PRACTICAL TIPS FOR OLDER SIBLINGS
>
> - **Start the bond early.** Encourage your toddler to talk to the bump, stroke it gently or sing to the baby while you're pregnant. It builds familiarity before the baby even arrives.
> - **Practise 'gentle'.** Use toys, dolls or even the bump to teach the idea of gentle hands. When baby comes, the word is already part of their vocabulary.
> - **Keep them included.** Let older siblings help in small, safe ways once the baby is here – passing you wipes, choosing an outfit or singing a lullaby. Feeling involved helps them feel important, not pushed aside.
> - **Protect their special time.** Even 10 minutes of undivided attention each day can reassure a toddler that they haven't lost you. Let them choose the activity, so it feels truly theirs.
> - **Use positive language.** Talk about the baby as 'our baby' or 'your baby brother/sister' to create a sense of ownership and pride.
> - **Expect big feelings.** Some regression (like wanting a bottle again or acting out) is normal. It's their way of

THE SECOND TRIMESTER

adjusting, not a sign of failure. Meet it with patience where you can.
- **The first meeting matters.** If possible, let your toddler meet the baby without lots of people around, so they have space to process it. Some parents like to have a 'gift from the baby' ready for the sibling – a small toy or book can make that first hello a little sweeter.

'OH, THAT'S NORMAL' . . . UNTIL IT'S NOT

Throughout pregnancy, you'll mention symptoms you're experiencing, and chances are, someone will respond with, *Oh yeah, that's normal.* Most of the time, they're right – until they're not. I've seen so many women get dismissed with a casual *That's normal* without any real explanation of when it stops being normal and becomes cause for concern. So let's talk about it. Here are some common pregnancy symptoms that many women experience throughout pregnancy, what makes them *actually* normal, and – more importantly – when I want you to stroll, walk, waddle or whatever you've got to do, straight to get checked out.

1. Swelling: Normal Puff or Red Flag?

   I have a theory – some babies hear us complaining about the water bill and decide to make sure we *retain* every last drop. Mild swelling in the feet, ankles and hands during your pregnancy? Completely normal. It happens because your body is holding onto extra fluid. What's *not* normal is sudden or severe swelling, especially in your face or hands. This could be a sign of pre-eclampsia, a pregnancy-related high blood pressure condition that needs medical attention.

2. **When a Headache Is More Than Just a Headache**
It's normal to have occasional headaches during pregnancy, thanks to hormones flying up and down, dehydration (especially if you can't keep anything down) or fatigue – because, again, you may not be able to keep anything down. What's *not* normal are persistent or severe headaches that don't go away with rest, paracetamol or hydration, especially if they come with blurred vision or swelling. These could be signs of high blood pressure or pre-eclampsia and need to be checked out.

3. **Pregnancy Back Pain: When to Stretch and When to Call the Doctor**
Your body isn't just housing your organs any more – it's now accommodating a whole baby, a placenta (aka baby's checked-in luggage) and amniotic fluid. That's a *lot* to carry. So, mild to moderate back pain caused by your growing belly, posture shifts and relaxin is totally normal. What's *not* normal? Severe back pain. But since pain thresholds vary, let's be more specific. If your back pain is sudden, one-sided or radiates down your legs, it could be a sign of a

THE SECOND TRIMESTER

kidney infection, preterm labour or even a herniated disc. In that case, don't wait it out – get checked.

4. **Pregnancy Discharge: The Good, The Bad and The 'Go Get Checked'**
   Even outside of pregnancy, discharge is a constant. Our vaginas are always working overtime. But during pregnancy? It's vaginal discharge, pro max edition. If it's clear or white with a mild smell, it's normal. Let's be real – it's *not* meant to smell like roses, so don't expect it to. What's *not* normal? Discharge that's green, yellow, has a strong foul smell or comes as a sudden gush of fluid. These could be signs of an infection, waters breaking early or preterm labour. If that happens, it's time to check in with your midwife or doctor.

5. **Your Baby's Activity: When a Quiet Day is Too Quiet**
   Just like us, babies have active days and slower days. It's completely normal for there to be variations in your baby's kicks. Some days they'll be having a party in there, other days they'll be a little more chilled. What's *not* normal? A noticeable drop or complete stop in movement after 28 weeks. If that happens, get checked ASAP. When it comes to foetal movement, it's always better to be safe than sorry.

6. **Breathlessness: Baby's Pressure vs. a Real Problem**
   Not only are you housing a human, but your *real estate* is expanding – so it's no surprise that breathing can feel a little harder, especially in the third trimester

when the baby starts pressing against your diaphragm (see page 136). What's *not* normal? Sudden, severe breathlessness, chest pain or dizziness. These could be signs of a blood clot (pulmonary embolism) or a heart issue, and that's not something to brush off. If you feel anything off, get checked.

7. **Pelvic Pressure: Normal or a Warning Sign?**

   As the baby drops lower in the third trimester, (see page 134) some pelvic pressure is completely normal. It's just your body getting ready for the big day. What's *not* normal? Intense pressure or the unsettling feeling that the baby is about to 'fall out' before full term. This could be a sign of preterm labour or cervical incompetence, and it's worth getting checked, ma'am.

8. **Braxton Hicks or Something More? Know the Difference**

   Occasional, irregular belly tightening that disappears with rest or hydration? That's just your uterus doing practice drills (see also page 135). What's *not* normal? Contractions that are regular, painful and don't ease up. If they start before 37 weeks, they could be a sign of preterm labour – and that's something you want to get checked *immediately.*

9. **Throwing Up? Fine. Throwing Up Everything? Not Fine.**

   Nausea and vomiting? Blame hCG. This pregnancy hormone is a sign that your baby is thriving – but it also means you might spend a lot of time with your head in the toilet. What's *not* normal? Vomiting so much that you feel completely drained, weak and start losing electrolytes. That's when 'normal' stops being normal and starts being a problem. If that happens, it's time to get checked.

10. **When Itching Isn't Just an Itch**

    A little skin itching as your belly stretches? Annoying, but totally normal. What's *not* normal? Severe itching, especially on your hands and feet, with no rash in sight. This could be a sign of intrahepatic cholestasis of pregnancy (ICP), a liver condition that affects bile flow and can increase the risk of complications. If you notice this, don't just assume it's 'one of those pregnancy things' – get checked.

CLOSING THE SECOND TRIMESTER

That's the second trimester, folks. What I want you to take out of this trimester is the reminder that you are learning as you go. You are getting to know your baby, your body and yourself in new ways. The second trimester often builds confidence, but it can also bring new uncertainties - especially as you start looking ahead to the third trimester and the reality of birth. If you find yourself worrying about what is to come, that does not mean you are unprepared. It means you are human.

I'M PREGNANT ... NOW WHAT?

The third trimester will ask different things of you – more rest, more patience and sometimes more flexibility as plans shift. But for now, know that the ground you have covered in these past few months is laying the foundation for everything to come.

SECOND TRIMESTER CHECKLIST

Here are some things you might want to tick off before heading into the third trimester:

- Book and attend your mid-pregnancy (20-week) scan.
- Start thinking about your birth preferences and jotting them down.
- If you want to attend antenatal classes, look into dates and book ahead.
- Begin discussing maternity leave plans with your employer.
- If you have older children, gently start preparing them for a new sibling.
- Look into childcare options if you will need them after the baby arrives.
- Keep up with routine blood tests, blood pressure checks and any extra scans offered.
- Consider practical purchases – maternity clothes that feel comfortable or the bigger baby items like a car seat.

THE SECOND TRIMESTER

- Keep nourishing yourself with balanced meals, hydration and rest where possible.
- Continue connecting with your baby – talk, sing or simply place your hand on your bump.

Remember, this checklist is not about doing everything perfectly or all at once.

PART 3

THE THIRD TRIMESTER

THE HOME STRETCH

Welcome to the third trimester, the land of 'when are you due?' over and over again. The land of trying to sleep – emphasis on the trying. The time when things start to feel *real*. You catch yourself in the mirror and laugh, remembering when you thought your bump was massive in the first and second trimesters – that little belly you kept imagining was huge, forever checking your side profile in front of the mirror – but yeah, *this* is the bump.

This is also when the questions get louder – on the outside *and* inside. Birth starts to feel closer, and so does the fear. The what-ifs. The birth anxiety that creeps in, even when you're doing everything 'right'. This is where we talk about all of that, because pretending it's not there doesn't make it go away.

I'M PREGNANT ... NOW WHAT?

It's the season of pressure – from yourself, from others. The pressure to have the *perfect* birth plan, and we'll talk about how to create one that actually works for *you* – one that holds space for flexibility, and one that doesn't crumble under expectations.

We'll also get into the physical bits, like the back pain that makes you want to throw your entire spine in the bin. The discomfort that creeps into your everyday. The body that feels like it's not yours any more, but is doing something *so* huge it almost deserves a round of applause every morning.

And beyond all that, how do you start preparing your *mind* for when your baby arrives? Conversations with your birth partner and your family, like: *when* do you want visitors? What kind of support feels good? How do you begin setting boundaries around the questions, the noise and the people that come with this season?

I say all this with my whole chest, because it's the small, intentional things now that can shift your whole experience later.

Let's talk about it all.

COUNTDOWNS AND EXPECTATIONS

The third trimester is about getting comfortable being uncomfortable. You're rolling from side to side like a rotisserie chicken, trying to sleep, trying to get comfy, trying not to cry when you drop something on the floor. The physical discomforts are real. But there's another type of discomfort that's just as important to face: the conversations.

This is the season where you've got to get comfortable having *uncomfortable* conversations. Boundaries don't just appear after birth – you start building them now. Conversations with your birth partner, your family, your friends. Setting expectations. Making it clear what support looks like for you. That kind of emotional preparation can make a *huge* difference to your labour and postnatal experience.

From what I've seen in my midwifery experience, and from what I've seen over and over again with other pregnant mummies, this one thing can be a real game-changer: stop telling everyone your exact due date. Everyone who *needs* to know already knows: your healthcare team, your close circle, your birth partner. What tends to happen is, once you hit that date, the messages start flooding in: *Any news? Is baby here yet? Still pregnant?*

And that constant questioning? It's not harmless. Psychologically, it puts you on a timer. It can make you feel like you're running late, like your body is behind schedule, when in reality, it's doing exactly what it's meant to. And here's the important part: when you feel that pressure, your adrenaline levels rise. And adrenaline? *Adrenaline hates oxytocin.* Oxytocin is the hormone that helps get labour going, strengthens your contractions and allows you to birth your baby. If your adrenaline's up, oxytocin struggles. So the more pressure you feel, the more your body can stall.

That's why these conversations matter. They don't have to be confrontational. This isn't a book about fighting your family or cutting people off. It could be as simple as saying, 'I read something interesting in this book. It said too many countdown messages can actually stress mums out and delay labour.'

Say it light. Say it with a smile. Make it a conversation, not a confrontation. If you're not up for saying anything directly, close to your due date, stop picking up every phone call. Train people now that you're not glued to your phone. That way, when you actually go quiet, it doesn't feel suspicious. And when you do pick up and they ask, just say, 'Yep, still here. All good.'

But listen, if you're the type of person who *loves* a countdown, who wants to post '10 days to go!' – go for it. Do what feels good for *you*. The key thing is that you're not suffering in silence or feeling cornered by pressure.

PHYSICAL SYMPTOMS AND DISCOMFORT

Let me run you through some of the most common physical symptoms that tend to show up in the third trimester. This is the point in pregnancy where your body is doing *everything*. Carrying the weight, preparing to birth and quite frankly, falling apart in ways that deserve acknowledgement.

Let's start with **back pain and pelvic pressure**. We've covered it before, but it's worth mentioning again, because

THE THIRD TRIMESTER

for some of you, this is not just a dull ache – it's serious. The kind of discomfort that makes getting out of bed feel like a gym session. The kind that stops you mid-step. And in some cases, it goes beyond general pregnancy aches. There's a condition called **Symphysis Pubis Dysfunction (SPD)**, and it's not rare. That's when the ligaments holding your pelvic bones together loosen too much, too early, which can cause sharp pain in your pubic area, groin, hips or even thighs. It is not something to 'just put up with'. If that sounds like you, speak to your midwife or doctor. Physiotherapy, pelvic support belts and pain relief are things that can help. SPD does not harm your baby, but it can have a big impact on you. For most women, the symptoms ease after birth as the hormones settle and the pelvis gradually stabilises again. But for some, especially if it was very severe in pregnancy, discomfort can continue into the postnatal period. That is why getting help early matters it can make recovery smoother and reduce the chances of long-term pain.

Then we've got **Braxton Hicks contractions**, which get more common and noticeable in this trimester. These are sometimes called 'practice' or 'false' contractions, and I just need to say this: there is *nothing false* about the pain some of you feel with them. Some tightenings are just that, but others come with cramping, backache and emotional exhaustion because they keep happening and going *nowhere*.

The main difference between Braxton Hicks and true labour contractions is that Braxton Hicks usually stay the same in intensity and don't get closer together over time.

Real contractions? They build. They increase. They come for you in waves. The hard bit is the *mental toll*, because when your body keeps throwing out signals and nothing happens, it can make you feel like your body's failing or confused. It's not. It's just gearing up.

Now, **swelling and puffiness**. You've probably started noticing that your feet don't fit into your old shoes and your hands feel like they've been inflated. That's because your body is holding onto a lot more fluid now and your growing uterus is putting pressure on veins that help return blood to your heart. When that flow slows down, fluid pools in your lower limbs and boom – sausage toes. Puffy ankles. Rings that don't fit any more. Your body's trying, but it's a lot to carry.

Same goes for **shortness of breath**. You could be doing *nothing*, literally just lying in bed, and feel like you've just sprinted. Your uterus is now pushing up against your diaphragm, the muscle that helps your lungs expand. Less space for your lungs means less air intake. This is common and expected. If you're suddenly finding it hard to breathe, or you can't speak in full sentences or it comes on out of nowhere, *that* is a red flag. That's when you need to get seen. Otherwise, the breathlessness that creeps in slowly and consistently? That's third trimester life.

Now let me give **urination** its moment. Yes, I've mentioned it *too many times* in this book. And yes, I'm going to keep mentioning it. As constant as urination is in pregnancy, is exactly how constant my references to it are going to be. You could pee, stand up and need to pee again. You

THE THIRD TRIMESTER

plan your outings around toilets. You hesitate to sneeze. You're up every hour in the night. It's not just a mild inconvenience – it's your new lifestyle. And while it's annoying for me to keep talking about it, it's even more annoying for you to be living it, so I will keep bringing it up for you. Again and again and again.

And that's the truth about the third trimester. Your body is working overtime. Every symptom, every puff of breath, every trip to the loo is a reminder that you are carrying life *and* being stretched to your limits.

There's a whole host of other symptoms you may experience, but I don't want this book to become one of those 'here's every single thing that could possibly happen in your body' guides. That's not the vibe. This isn't a pregnancy horror story collection. It's not a 'get ready for all this mess' manual. But at the same time, I'd be lying if I said third trimester didn't come with some extra bits that *can* show up for some people, such as:

- leaky boobs
- intense heartburn
- itchy skin
- pelvic pain
- haemorrhoids
- constipation
- hot flushes
- clumsiness
- pins and needles in extremities

- vivid dreams
- varicose veins

But let me tell you why I won't try to give you an exhaustive list of everything that could ever happen to a pregnant body. I could study pregnancy for *hundreds* of years and still not capture every single symptom a woman might experience. Honestly, one woman once asked me, 'Is it weird that my thumb looks a bit bigger?' And I remember thinking, *You know what? At this point, nothing surprises me any more.* The body does wild, wonderful, strange things in pregnancy, and not all of it fits into a textbook. So if you feel something that isn't mentioned in this book, please don't panic. It doesn't mean you're broken or imagining things. It just means your experience is *yours*. I couldn't possibly name every symptom. I'm not here to tell you what's *definitely* going to happen. I'm here to help you spot the common stuff, prepare for what might happen, and give you enough knowledge that you feel informed, not overwhelmed.

Because like I always say – ignorance isn't bliss when it comes to pregnancy.

SLEEP (OR LACK THEREOF)

Imagine this. You've finally found that one position that feels just right. You've built a fortress of pillows, adjusted your leg angle, supported your bump, placed one arm under,

THE THIRD TRIMESTER

one arm over, even tilted your neck like it's some sacred yoga pose. Your breathing's steady. You're still. You can feel sleep brushing past you. And then . . . you need to wee.

So you drag yourself out of your masterpiece of a position, waddle to the toilet for the fifteenth time, and by the time you're back in bed, everything feels off again. Your hip aches. Baby's kicked up a storm. You start to think about what time it is, what you haven't packed yet, what contractions might feel like, whether the hospital bag needs more snacks and whether you even know what you're doing.

This is third trimester sleep. It's not even like you're awake because you want to be. You're *tired*. Like, genuinely, completely, deep-in-your-bones *tired*. And that's what makes it worse. There is *nothing* – and I mean *nothing* – more frustrating than being absolutely exhausted and still not being able to sleep. Your body's done for the day. Your mind wants to switch off. But between your bladder, baby movements, dodgy hip and overthinking, there's just no peace.

People love to give advice. 'Try relaxing.' 'Have a warm bath.' 'Read a book before bed.' I mean, sure, those things might help someone somewhere, but let's not act like a cup of camomile tea is going to undo the fact that your entire body is shifting, your hormones are all over the place and your brain is in survival mode.

Some of it, yes, is physical. You're heavier. Your centre of gravity is off. There's a small human pushing into your ribs while your organs are being shuffled around like furniture. Then there's the classic: 'Don't sleep on your back.'

I'M PREGNANT ... NOW WHAT?

That one's backed by science. When you lie flat on your back in late pregnancy, your growing uterus can compress a major vein called the **inferior vena cava**. That's the one that carries blood from your lower body back to your heart. If it's compressed for too long, it can reduce blood flow to both you *and* baby. So we say to lie on your side, preferably your left, but your right is okay too. Your body will usually tell you what it likes. Just know that there's a reason you keep waking up the moment you lie flat for too long. It's not in your head.

But the other side of insomnia – the side that isn't about pillows or positions – is the *mental stuff*. The spiral of thoughts that hits you as soon as the room goes dark. Let's not pretend it's all rational. Sometimes the thoughts make sense, sometimes they don't. Sometimes you're crying because you saw a nappy ad at 1 a.m. Sometimes you're up googling 'Can I eat crunchy peanut butter in labour?' just in case. It's not even funny when it's happening, but the next day you look back and think, *This pregnancy thing is unhinged*.

Now, some mummies have said certain things have helped them. This is all down to personal preference and what works best for you. Some mums mentioned:

- Hypnobirthing tracks that talk you down into a relaxed state.
- The kind of calming gospel music that makes your body feel like it's exhaling.
- Soft Quran recitations that settle the spirit.

- Guided meditations that take you through every part of your body like a mental scan.
- Building that full-body pillow fortress with zero shame – back, belly, knees, ankles, neck.
- Warm showers.
- White noise.
- Lavender oils.
- Putting the phone down and forcing yourself to *just lie still* for a bit, even if sleep doesn't come straight away.
- Journalling what's on your mind to stop your brain from playing ping-pong all night.

None of these are promises. None of them are guaranteed. Trust me, if I ever find the formula that works for *everyone*, I'll be a millionaire. I'll be selling sleep kits with a smug smile and a silk robe. But until then, all I can do is tell you the truth: insomnia in the third trimester is *rough*. It's layered. It's not just about being uncomfortable; it's about carrying the physical weight of your baby *and* the emotional weight of becoming a mum. So if you're tossing and turning, and nothing seems to help, know that you're not alone in this. You're part of a whole world of mummies doing exactly the same thing at 3:47 a.m.

THE EMOTIONAL MENTAL LOAD

Let's get into the part that people love to skip over when talking about pregnancy: the emotional bit. The mental load. The 'what's going on in my head and heart' part. Because as much as your body is doing the most right now, your *mind* is right there doing overtime too.

Let's start with **fear of labour and birth anxiety**. For some mummies, this shows up right from the first trimester. Especially if it's your first pregnancy, as you're facing the fear of the unknown. You've probably watched videos online, heard stories from friends, seen some chaotic TikToks and suddenly your brain is like, *How am I meant to survive this?* You've never done it before, so of course it feels big. That's normal.

But I've also seen this fear show up in people who've done it before, and you'd think, surely they'd feel confident, right? Not always. Sometimes it's because their last birth wasn't what they hoped for. Maybe it was traumatic. Maybe it was confusing. Maybe they just felt unseen in the process. Sometimes it's not even about past trauma – it's just the fact that every labour is different. Every baby is different. Everybody is different. You could do this 10 times and still feel a bit nervous about how it'll go. That's not a lack of strength – that's a completely human response to a massive event.

So how do you deal with the fear? The short answer: *talk*. Talk to someone. Talk to *anyone*. I honestly can't emphasise enough how important it is to have someone in pregnancy that you can open up to. A friend, your partner, a midwife, a therapist, someone in a class. The silence is where fear grows legs. When you hold everything in, it gets heavier.

THE THIRD TRIMESTER

When you say it out loud, even if it doesn't fix anything, it *shifts* something. Sometimes the moment you say it, you realise it's not as big as it felt in your head. Sometimes, the other person gives you language for something you couldn't explain yourself. Either way, don't keep it in.

Something people often gloss over is **anticipatory grief**. That sense of mourning the version of you that's about to change. Sometimes, especially for first-time mums, it gets painted over with 'everything is new and magical' but even magic has its costs. For others, especially if it's baby number two or three, it might feel more complex. Maybe you've just found yourself again. Maybe you've started going out again, feeling sexy again, chasing your dreams again. And now ... it's all about to change again.

My friend Lola had a baby and then got pregnant again just after her first turned one. She'd just started to get herself back – going to the gym, feeling more like herself, easing into a bit of balance. And then, boom. Pregnant again. She told me how hard it was to mentally prepare, not just for doing it all over again, but for the fact that it would be different this time. She grieved the energy she had the first time around, the new-mum excitement, the space to prepare emotionally. And one thing that really stayed with me was when she said, 'It's the fact that this next baby won't get the same version of me.' That hit. Because it's not just about what *you* lose – it's the guilt of wondering if your next child will feel it too. That feeling of, 'Will I have enough to give?' That's a grief in itself.

And if you've never heard anyone say it before, I want you to hear it now: you're not weird or ungrateful for feeling it. You're human. You're transitioning. And grief doesn't mean regret – it means you're acknowledging change. It means you care.

I want to say this clearly: *I wish this didn't have to be part of the process.* I *wish* motherhood didn't come with a sense of loss, but for many women, it does. And that doesn't make you selfish or ungrateful. It makes you honest. And while motherhood will absolutely change you, I don't believe it should erase you. There *will* be a shift in who you are, but that doesn't mean you disappear. You don't have to become unrecognisable to become a good mum. So if you're grieving a bit while also preparing for joy, that's okay. That's real.

WAYS TO HOLD ON TO YOURSELF AFTER BIRTH

- Keep something that is just for you – a hobby, journalling or a ritual that reminds you of who you are outside of motherhood.
- Protect small moments of time – even 10 minutes a day to rest, breathe or do something that brings you joy.
- Ask for help and accept it. Let partners, family or friends step in so you can have a break.

THE THIRD TRIMESTER

- Be honest about what you need – even if you aren't sure. Saying 'I don't know what I need, but I know I need support' is enough.
- Reframe self-care as essential, not indulgent. The more cared-for you are, the more present you can be for your baby.

And finally, let's talk about that feeling of being **'done' but also not ready**. That strange little space where you're emotionally cooked but mentally not quite prepared. You could be someone who's done everything; you've packed the bag, set up the cot, read all the books, bought the snacks and still feel like you're not ready. Or you could be like me: *very* lastminute.com. You're still working out what time means. And the car seat? Yeah, it's still in the box.

That unsure feeling? It's not a sign you won't cope. It's just the unknown talking. So shift your focus. Think about the moment your baby's on your chest. The way they'll curl into you. The way you'll meet for the first time after all these months of wondering. That's what's coming. That's what you hold onto.

And please hear this – your baby isn't going to care if you forgot to buy a second changing mat or didn't label your hospital bag. I've never once said to my mum, 'Wow, can't believe you didn't get that car seat sorted on time.' That's not what matters.

PUTTING A SPOTLIGHT ON MATERNAL MENTAL HEALTH

Let's address mental health **properly**.

One of my friends called me once, clearly overwhelmed. She said, 'Why does nobody talk about mental health in pregnancy?' And it stuck with me. She felt like she was waiting for her feelings to feel justified, like she couldn't fully admit she was struggling because she hadn't had the baby yet. Like the only time you're allowed to feel not-okay is in the postnatal period. I had to remind her, and I'll remind you too: **you don't have to wait until the baby's here to be overwhelmed.**

The truth is, we don't talk enough about mental health during pregnancy. I know that sounds wild, coming from someone who lives in the maternity space. But even as a midwife, I don't always get to meet mums in the thick of it while they're pregnant. And yet when I do, the stories pour out. The exhaustion. The intrusive thoughts. The moments where they felt disconnected, anxious or flat – but told themselves they had to keep it moving because 'everything's fine on the scan'.

There's research now that tells us what many of us already knew deep down – mental health issues can show up in pregnancy just as much as they do after birth, and often they become more prominent in the

THE THIRD TRIMESTER

third trimester. The pressure builds. Your body feels foreign. You're running on empty. There's excitement, yes, but also fear. Uncertainty. Guilt about not being as 'grateful' as you think you're supposed to be. Add that to a poor night's sleep (again), a back that's screaming, and a well-meaning friend asking, 'How's maternity leave?' like it's a spa retreat, and you've got the perfect cocktail for mental overload.

I don't want to brush past this with a casual 'it's normal' either. Yes, there are moments where worry is a natural part of preparing for birth, but there's a line, and if you feel like you're sinking, if you feel like your thoughts are louder than they should be, if you're crying more days than you're not, if you're scared and don't know why, you deserve support. Not judgement. Not silence. Support.

Talk to someone. Your midwife. Your GP. Your friend. A therapist. You don't need to suffer in silence to 'earn' your motherhood badge. You're already doing the work.

My friend was right to ask. It reminded me that we cannot afford to ignore mental health during pregnancy. The stories are real. The feelings are valid. And just because it's common doesn't mean it should go unspoken. Because like I always say: ignorance isn't bliss when it comes to pregnancy – and that includes your mental well-being.

THIRD TRIMESTER APPOINTMENTS: WHAT TO EXPECT

By the time you reach the third trimester, your appointments tend to feel a bit more regular. There are more blood pressure checks, more belly measurements, more chats about birth. But for a lot of mummies, this can be the part where it all starts to blur. Some feel like nothing is really happening. Others feel like *everything* is happening. Depending on your pregnancy, you could be floating through with just a few check-ins, or suddenly booked in for scan after scan after scan. Let's break that down a bit.

Let's talk about **growth scans** first. Now, not everyone will have one of these in the third trimester. In fact, if you've had a straightforward pregnancy, you probably won't be booked in for any more routine scans after your 20-week anomaly scan. That's it for the official NHS schedule. But if there's something your team wants to monitor more closely, like baby's growth, the fluid around baby or the position of the placenta, then you might be sent for one or more growth scans.

And when I say 'monitor', I mean exactly that. It's not always because something is *wrong*. Sometimes it's just a precaution, or a check to be sure. For example, if baby's bump measurement is looking a little smaller or larger than expected, they might want to check the weight more accurately via ultrasound. Or if there's a concern about too much fluid or too little fluid around baby, they'll have a closer look. Or maybe baby was breech at your last appointment and they want to see if they've turned.

But if your pregnancy has been nice and uneventful (and long may it stay that way), you might not get another NHS scan unless there's a specific reason. That doesn't mean you *can't* have one – it just means it's not routine. If you want the reassurance or just want another look at baby, you're always welcome to book a private scan. Some mummies love having those extra peeks, even just to ease their mind before labour. Others don't feel the need. It's all about what feels good for you.

Now, let's move on to **Group B Strep** (GBS). This one can cause a lot of anxiety, especially when people start googling. So let's calm that down and walk through it clearly. Group B Strep is a type of bacteria that some women carry in their vagina or rectum. It's not a sexually transmitted infection, and it's not dangerous for you during pregnancy, but in *rare* cases, it can be passed to baby during labour and cause an infection. The good news is, if we *know* you're carrying it, we can do something about it.

Some hospitals will routinely test for GBS in late pregnancy, usually around 35–37 weeks. In other areas, it's only tested if there's a reason, like if it was found in your urine earlier on, or if you've had a baby previously affected by GBS. If you do test positive, please don't panic. It doesn't mean you've done anything wrong. It doesn't mean your baby is automatically at risk. What we do is simple: once your waters break or you go into labour, we start you on IV antibiotics. That's it. The antibiotics help prevent the bacteria from crossing over to baby. It's what we call a **prophylactic measure**, meaning it's done to reduce risk before anything even happens. So rather than being scared of a positive result, think of it this way: the fact that we know means we can protect your baby.

BEST-LAID PLANS

Now, onto one of the biggest pressure points of the third trimester: **birth planning**. Or as I prefer to call it, *birth preferences.*

Here's the thing. I'm still not 100 per cent sure how I feel about the phrase 'birth plan'. Because planning can sound so rigid. So final. So *goal-oriented*. And birth? Birth doesn't always follow the plan. But I *am* a huge believer in *not walking into your labour clueless*. You don't need to have every outcome mapped, but you *do* need to be informed. You need to know your options. You need to understand what's available to you and how to speak up when things change.

A birth plan isn't a to-do list. It's not about ticking off achievements. It's not about writing, *I want a vaginal birth with no pain relief,* and then feeling like a failure if it doesn't happen. It's about expressing your *preferences* while staying open to the fact that things might shift. It's saying: 'I'd prefer not to have pain relief, but if I feel overwhelmed, I'm open to an epidural.' Or: 'I'd love a vaginal birth, but I understand that if baby's heartbeat drops, I may need a C-section.' It's about flexibility. It's about being informed and adaptable at the same time. The most disappointing thing that could happen would be to carry your baby for months, go through everything pregnancy has thrown at you, and then get to the finish line feeling like you 'failed' because your birth didn't go to plan. You didn't fail. You *birthed*.

I've said this before and I'll say it again: there's no science behind it, but I've seen it time and time again – mummies who come in saying, 'I'm not having this, I'm not having that, I'm not having that,' somehow end up needing *all of that*. It's not about jinxing it. But it's a good reminder to stay open, because when you're open, you can adapt, and when you're informed, you can make decisions with confidence.

So educate yourself. Learn about all the options – water birth, induction, epidural, gas and air, home birth, caesarean, TENS machines, whatever's out there. Know about the interventions, the risks, the benefits. Not to prepare for every possible path, but so that whatever path *you* end up on, you walk it knowing your rights, your voice and your power.

Because here's the truth: it's not the *type* of birth that gives you power. It's the fact that you made **informed choices**. That's where the real power lies.

Birth Plan Checklist

When you're putting your birth plan together, think about:

- What kind of birth you'd like (vaginal, water birth, planned caesarean, etc.).
- What pain relief options you'd like to try (and which ones you'd prefer to avoid).
- Whether you'd like to be asked regularly about pain relief or only if you bring it up.
- Who you want in the room with you (partner, friend, doula, etc.).
- Whether you're comfortable with students being present.
- How you'd like the space to feel (lights, music, scents, privacy).
- How you'd like to deliver the placenta (naturally or with an injection).
- Whether you'd like immediate skin-to-skin contact after birth.
- Your preferences for feeding (breast, bottle, or combination).
- Who should cut the cord — or if you want delayed cord clamping.
- What you'd like to happen if things don't go to plan (for example, if a caesarean becomes necessary).

THE THIRD TRIMESTER

HOSPITAL BAG PACKING

Let me first say: how long you'll stay in hospital really depends. If your birth is straightforward and there are no complications, you might be home within six to 24 hours. Some countries discharge people even sooner. On the flip side, if you or baby need monitoring, you might be in for a little while. So this is a **general guide** to help you feel prepared – not a 'you must bring this all' list. And let's be real: if you forget something, chances are the hospital isn't too far. Someone can run back home. Here's what you *actually* need.

For Mummy:

- Your hospital notes (don't leave them on the kitchen table . . . I've seen it too many times).
- Comfortable bras (wireless, soft, maybe nursing-friendly).
- Two packs of super absorbent sanitary pads.
- Knickers (preferably disposable or old ones you don't care about).
- A wash bag with your basics (toothbrush, toothpaste, lip balm, deodorant, etc.).
- One large towel + one face towel.
- A handheld fan or water spray (trust me, labour sweat is a different kind of sweat).
- Front-opening or loose-fitted nighties (ideally two – one for labour, one post-birth).

- A loose outfit for going home. (Don't pack your pre-pregnancy jeans. Just don't.)
- Healthy snacks (fruit/nut bars, sweets, nuts – labour is hungry work).
- Extra pillows (NHS is broke).
- Any medication you're currently taking.
- A hot water bottle or heat pack.
- Phone charger (ideally with a long cable).
- Something for your brain: book, playlist, podcast, Netflix download.

For Baby:

- A few baby vests and sleepsuits (three).
- A hat and blanket (three).
- Nappies and wipes (one pack).
- Cotton wool balls (some hospitals prefer it for newborn bottoms).
- Bottles and pre-made formula (if you plan to combo or formula feed).
- If you're planning to breastfeed and have harvested colostrum, bring that with you too (keep it in the freezer, and once you get to the birthing unit, give it to your midwife to store it).

Now let me pause and say this because it matters: **if you're planning to breastfeed, but you haven't harvested colostrum,** or you weren't able to, *you are still doing great.* When baby arrives, it's a huge shock to your system. And sometimes, the milk doesn't flow right away. My biggest worry is a new mummy feeling panicked at 3 a.m., with a hungry baby crying and no backup plan. So please hear me: **bringing a bottle of pre-made milk 'just in case' does not make you the devil**. It doesn't mean you've failed. It doesn't mean you'll use it. But sometimes, it's like that thing you don't think you'll need – but when you do, and it's not there? The stress hits different. Having it on hand can save you from that panic. And if you don't need it? Great. But if you do, you'll be so glad it's there. It's not about replacing your breastfeeding journey – it's about protecting your peace of mind.

For Your Birth Partner:

They're not just 'there to help'. They're part of the team. Here's what they should pack:

- Phone and charger (with space for pics/videos).
- Snacks and drinks (you don't want a hangry partner in the delivery room).
- A change of clothes (especially if it's a long labour or they stay overnight).
- Toiletries (deodorant, toothbrush – don't let the room smell like stress).
- Cash/card for car park, vending machines, emergency snacks.
- Headphones.

- List of your birth preferences (on phone or printed).
- Water spray/fan (for you!).

PREPPING YOUR VILLAGE

Let's talk about support – not just who says they'll help, but who actually will. Now's the time to start thinking about what you'll need once baby arrives. For some people, that might be a full house, constant visitors, someone to talk to, someone to hold the baby while they nap. For others, it might mean silence, space, a few days to find their feet before anyone else enters the room. Whichever one you are, both are valid. You just need to start talking about it now.

It's okay to say, 'We'll let you know when we're ready for visitors,' and mean it. It's also okay to say, 'We'd love your help with dinners or cleaning for the first few days.' Whatever your version of support looks like, claim it. The more you prep now, the less tension or awkwardness you'll feel later. This is your space, your recovery, your new rhythm. You deserve to feel safe and supported.

The phrase, 'it takes a village' didn't come from nowhere. It's not just something people say – it's rooted in truth. I've seen so many videos and posts with people writing passive notes to their families or sticking messages on the front door about visitors, and I'll be honest, I don't like it. Not because boundaries aren't important, but because I think a lot of it comes down to how we say things and whether we communicated them clearly in the first place. When you've already set the tone and been honest about what you need, it doesn't have to turn into a performance.

If you're someone lucky enough to have access to a village, use it. Don't shut it out trying to be overly independent. I know there's a narrative these days that you've got to do it all alone to prove something, but that's not how we were made. We were designed to lean on each other. Support is needed. And I've spoken to so many mums, even the most organised, list-loving, Type A mums, who've said they thought they had it all covered until they realised they didn't. When the time came, they didn't know how to ask for help. So start now. Be clear, be kind and remember that boundaries and support can exist at the same time.

If you've already got a little one or a furry family member, then you already know: baby isn't just a shift for you – it's a shift for them too. Siblings can feel unsure, pets might act differently, and it's all totally normal. The trick is to find gentle ways to fold them into the transition. You don't have to stage some big dramatic moment. Just small conversations, little bits of involvement. Let your older child feel seen. Let them help in whatever way makes sense.

You don't need to do it all perfectly. You just need to prepare in a way that feels manageable for you. Google might give you 101 tips and tricks, but what matters most is that everyone in your home feels a little more ready for the change, even if it's just by starting the conversation now.

I'M PREGNANT ... NOW WHAT?

MATERNITY LEAVE AND WORK PREPARATION

Whether you're employed or self-employed, now's the time to start putting things in place so you can actually *switch off*. Sort your handovers. Tie up loose ends. Set that out-of-office. Just let people know you're unavailable. You're not replying for a reason, and you don't need to feel guilty about that.

If you work for yourself, let your team, your clients or even your audience know what to expect. Communicate it clearly. Protect your time before baby comes, and especially when they arrive. I always tell people: don't be a Kat. Let me explain.

Kat is my manager. One time, I messaged her asking about something she had printed for me. Normal conversation. She calmly replied, 'I'll get back to you soon – I'm in labour, I think I'll be like 3cm!' As in, mid-contraction. Still trying to be responsive. Kat is brilliant, but please, don't be a Kat.

Be a Sade. My hairdresser had the most iconic maternity leave energy I've ever seen. I once DM'd her because I was ready to cut my hair into a full pixie. I was committed. But I was immediately hit with a sharp, automated response: 'I'm currently on maternity leave, not responding to DMs and not taking on any new clients at this time.' Lord knows I wanted that pixie cut badly – but I took it as a sign. I didn't need it. I still had my braids in. But the way that message came through? She was not playing.

So don't be a Kat. Be a Sade. Protect your peace, your time, and your uterus.

UNIQUE JOURNEYS FOR THE THIRD TRIMESTER

Not every pregnancy follows the textbook version and that's perfectly okay. For some, the third trimester comes with extra considerations, extra monitoring, or simply a different path to birth. Whether you've been told your pregnancy is 'high risk', you're planning a vaginal birth after a C-section, you're expecting twins (or more!), or you're navigating how your identity or background might shape your experience, this section is for you. It's all about understanding what makes your journey unique.

THE HIGH-RISK LABEL

Let's talk about the phrase *'high-risk pregnancy'*. I'm going to be honest – I'm not a huge fan of it. It sounds heavy, a bit medicalised, and almost like a warning sign stamped across someone's notes. But what it really means is that something in the pregnancy has crossed a certain line. Pregnancy has many of those invisible lines, and if something nudges slightly outside of what's expected, whether that's on a scan, in a blood test or based on previous medical history, that's when extra care is offered. The term 'high-risk' might sound like something is wrong, but it's often just the system saying: we're going to keep a closer eye on things. It's about prevention, not panic. Because what we know, we can support. What we don't know, we can't.

There are so many reasons why a pregnancy might be classed as high-risk, and I couldn't possibly name them all, but I can give you a feel for how that care might look if it happens.

Gestational diabetes: You may need to attend a diabetes clinic, be given a glucose monitor to check your blood sugar levels several times a day, and possibly be seen by a dietitian. You may need to adjust your diet or, in some cases, take medication or insulin. There would also be growth scans to check baby's size and amniotic fluid levels, since diabetes can affect both.

Pre-eclampsia: You might have your blood pressure monitored more frequently – sometimes at home with a monitor, sometimes through regular hospital visits. Blood tests and urine samples would become more frequent, and you may be asked to come in for CTG monitoring to track baby's movements and well-being. In some cases, this might mean being admitted to hospital for observation.

History of complications (e.g. haemorrhage, stillbirth, emergency C-section): You might be referred to a consultant-led team. You might be offered extra scans, earlier discussions about birth plans and access to specific clinics like a birth reflections clinic or a maternal medicine team who tailor care around previous experiences.

Sometimes, it's something picked up in a scan – maybe a concern about baby's heart, kidneys or something structural. In those cases, the woman may be referred to a foetal medicine unit, where more specialised assessments take place. Appointments might be longer, more frequent and involve multiple professionals – such as consultants, sonographers, midwives, paediatricians. The idea is not to bombard, but to inform and to plan ahead.

Care can include iron infusions for anaemia, injections for clotting disorders, medication adjustments for long-term health conditions like epilepsy, or simply more frequent monitoring if baby is measuring smaller or larger than expected. All of this to say – yes, the phrase 'high-risk' exists, but it doesn't mean that pregnancy is doomed or broken. What it means is that there's a different kind of attention. More eyes, more checks, more tools in place to help and protect both mother and baby.

You may not have any of these diagnoses, and I hope that's the case, but understanding what the care *can* look like is empowering. It helps remove the fear when someone throws the term around. It helps you understand that close monitoring is not the same as danger. It's a safety net. Because again: what we know, we can support. What we don't know, we can't.

VAGINAL BIRTH AFTER C-SECTION (VBAC)

Now, I try not to make this book the land of *my opinion, my opinion, my opinion* – that's not the vibe here. But I'd actually be doing a huge disservice if I stayed completely neutral on this one. Because the reality is – a lot of C-sections that are performed today? They aren't *always* necessary. There are far too many women who've told me they felt rushed, coerced or simply weren't given enough information before being taken into theatre.

With more and more people becoming informed, asking questions, and taking ownership over their births, we're seeing a rise in mummies who want to try for a VBAC, and I have to talk about it. Not because I want to scare you or because I think C-sections are bad – sometimes they are absolutely life-saving – but because I want you to understand that *you have options*, and VBAC is one of them.

So what does VBAC care look like? In most cases, it's recommended that VBACs happen in hospital settings. That's because there's a small risk of uterine rupture from the scar on the womb. I'm not here to hype that up or downplay it – it's just something your team will want to monitor closely. So yes, you'll likely be offered continuous monitoring during labour. You may be seen by both midwives and doctors throughout, and your baby's heartbeat will be tracked more regularly. VBACs aren't typically supported at home or in standalone midwifery-led units, because if intervention *was* needed, proximity to surgical care matters. But again, I'm not here to tell you what to do – I'm here to tell you what that care can look like so you're not caught off guard.

What you'll notice with VBAC care is that it's a little more watchful, a bit more hands-on. This is not because anyone assumes something will go wrong, but because it's better to be prepared. You might also hear conversations around how long labour is taking, how contractions are progressing, and whether any intervention might be needed.

There are certain things that can make a VBAC more likely to be successful: spontaneous labour (where your body goes into labour naturally), having had a vaginal birth before, even if it was before your caesarean, and how long ago your last surgery was. The baby's position and general pregnancy health also play a role. But hear me loud and clear: **you didn't fail if you want a VBAC and end up with another caesarean.**

At the end of the day, informed choices are what matter. Not the mode of birth. Not ticking a box. Not proving anything to anyone. When you understand your options, you move from being *told what to do* to *deciding what to do*.

BIRTHING WHILE BLACK

In the UK, Black women are currently three times more likely to die during pregnancy or childbirth than white women.[15] That statistic can sound terrifying, but it does not mean that one in three Black women will die.

Maternal mortality in the UK is still low overall. What it does mean is that there is a real inequality that cannot be ignored, and it is rooted in systemic issues – not in who you are as an individual, not in your worth, and not in whether you 'deserve' care.

So how do you navigate pregnancy knowing this? My biggest advice is to centre education and self-advocacy. Learn about your pregnancy, understand what is happening in your body, and don't be afraid to ask questions at every step. Ask for your test results and make sure you understand them. If you feel rushed in an appointment, say so. Let your provider know that you need more time, that you need things explained again or that you want to be more involved in decisions. You are entitled to that care.

It is important to remember this is not about needing only Black midwives or only Black doctors. This is not a problem that can be solved by individual providers. It is a systemic issue, and the most powerful thing you can do is make sure your voice is heard within that system. Advocate for the care you deserve, and never apologise for wanting to be fully seen, fully informed, and fully respected.

THE THIRD TRIMESTER

MULTIPLE BIRTHS

First of all, just know that I am absolutely obsessed with twin pregnancies. And triplets? Don't even tempt me – I might just move in with you. I still remember the very first twin pregnancy I looked after as a delivery midwife, and I was honestly fascinated. I'd be monitoring one baby, trying to get that perfect trace, and before I knew it – boom – baby's moved, or I'm picking up the same baby's heartbeat, and I'm like, *Wait, what the heck?!* It was a whole new world for me. Everything doubled; the scans, the paperwork (I was going to pass out), the monitoring. You really do realise just how much of a miracle it is to grow one baby, let alone two or more.

So let's talk about how third trimester care shifts a little when you're carrying twins or multiples – because this chapter is all about how things change in that final stretch.

Carrying more than one baby usually means **more appointments, more scans and closer monitoring** – not because something's wrong, but because you're doing double the work and your body is carrying double the load. You'll likely be having regular growth scans to track each baby's size, fluid levels and position. And depending on whether your babies share a placenta or have their own, you might be seen more frequently by a consultant-led team or referred to foetal medicine.

Let's get a little science-y for a second. One of the big reasons for this extra attention is the **increased risk of preterm labour**. That stretched uterus? It gets full quicker. There's more pressure on the cervix, more activity overall, so there's a higher chance of labour starting before 37 weeks. That doesn't mean it *will* happen, but we plan *just in case*. That could mean steroid injections to help the babies' lungs mature, or simply making sure your hospital bag is packed a bit earlier than usual. It's just about being ahead of the game.

Then there's the **logistics of delivery**. If Baby A is head-down and everything's looking good, a vaginal birth might still be very much on the cards, even with twins. Sometimes, especially if one or both babies are breech or there are other factors, your team might recommend a planned caesarean. Every twin pregnancy is different, and so is every care plan. This isn't about one rule for all – it's about **you**, your babies and what's safest and most supportive.

Just because there are more scans, more people in the room or more equipment doesn't mean you're not in control. On the day of delivery, it's a full house: **two midwives, two baby doctors**, sometimes even a third just in case. In fact, at my hospital, we literally use **Room 5**, the biggest room on the labour ward, for our twin mummies, because we know we are about to receive many guests. Always remember you can ask for updates and ask questions throughout – staying informed keeps you part of the picture, rather than feeling like things are just being done to you.

PART 4

THE BIG PUSH (LITERALLY)

WELCOME, BABY!

Okay, let me be real with you – I've *been waiting* to get to this chapter. This right here? This is *my jam*. My bread and butter. My everything. I've worked on labour wards for *years*, and I've seen and supported *hundreds* of births. I've held hands, wiped brows, cleaned vomit off mum, cleaned vomit off myself, given pep talks mid-contraction, and quietly whispered, 'You've got this,' when everything felt like too much. I've seen babies born to the sound of Afrobeats, gospel choirs, deep breathing, the Quran and even complete silence. One mum even made me play *Countdown* on the TV during her labour – I'm telling you, I've *seen it all*.

So if you're reading this with nerves, excitement, fear or all three – you're in the right place. This is where we get into the *real* stuff. The day your baby is born. So, deep breath. You're not alone. I'm here to guide you through every contraction, curveball and crowning moment (pun intended). Let's go – we've got a baby to meet.

STAGES OF LABOUR – BREAKING DOWN WHAT TO EXPECT AT EACH POINT

I know the movies make it seem like your waters break and you're pushing 10 minutes later, but real labour is not a Hollywood scene. It's a **process**, and that process can look very different depending on what baby number this is for you.

First-time mums, I'm sorry to say, but this can be a long journey. The **first stage** can take hours, days or even weeks in some cases. You'll hear stories of women who walk around 1cm for a whole week or more before things really kick off. Second-, third- or fourth-time mums, your body has already done this before, so things might move a bit quicker. Lucky you.

But whether you're on baby number one or baby number five, it's all normal. So let's break it down.

STAGE 1: EARLY LABOUR AND ACTIVE LABOUR

Early Labour can last forever. Your cervix is starting to dilate and efface (soften and thin out), but it can be a long process, especially if this is your first baby. Here's what you can expect:

THE BIG PUSH (LITERALLY)

- Contractions might be mild and irregular.
- You might feel a dull ache in your lower back or a tightening in your abdomen.
- You might lose your mucus plug or have a bloody show (a bit of blood-streaked mucus).
- Your waters might break, but this doesn't always happen in early labour.
- You might still be able to walk, talk and function relatively normally at this stage.

Active Labour is when things get real. Your contractions will get stronger, longer and closer together. Here's what to expect:

- Your cervix will dilate from around 4cm to 10cm.
- You'll probably find it harder to talk or walk through contractions.
- You might feel pressure in your lower back or pelvis.
- You might need to focus and breathe through each contraction.

STAGE 2: PUSHING AND BIRTH

All right, you're 10cm dilated, and now it's time to push.

- You may feel an overwhelming urge to bear down or push as your baby descends through the birth canal.

- Some women describe this stage as intense, but also a bit relieving because they feel like they're finally doing something.
- You might feel a burning or stretching sensation (often called the 'ring of fire') as baby crowns.
- This stage can be quick (especially if you've done this before) or it can take hours if it's your first baby.

STAGE 3: DELIVERY OF THE PLACENTA

Hey there, fun fact: you actually have to give birth twice. Yep. You've birthed your baby, but you still need to birth the placenta, which I like to call your baby's checked-in luggage.

Think of it like this: when you get off a plane, you still have to wait for your luggage at baggage claim. It's the same thing. Baby's out, but we're still waiting for their luggage. This stage can take anywhere from a few minutes to about an hour, depending on how you decide to birth the placenta.

You've got two main options:

- **Physiological Delivery** – when you wait for the placenta to come away naturally, without any injections. It can take a bit longer, but it's all about letting the body do its thing.

THE BIG PUSH (LITERALLY)

- **Active Management** – when you have a shot of syntocinon to speed things up. It encourages the uterus to contract and detach the placenta a bit faster.

You might feel some mild contractions as your uterus clamps down to push the placenta out, but it's usually not as intense as labour contractions.

The midwife will check the placenta to make sure it's all intact and that nothing has been left behind, because trust me, you don't want to be walking around with a bit of luggage left in the lounge.

STAGE 4: RECOVERY AND BONDING (GOLDEN HOUR)

This is the golden hour – that beautiful time when you and baby are finally together.

- You'll probably feel a rush of emotions, a bit of shock and a whole lot of relief.
- Your midwives will be checking to make sure you're stable, your bleeding is under control, and baby is feeding well.
- Skin-to-skin contact is encouraged if you and baby are both stable.
- This is the time for first feeds, snuggles and a whole lot of baby gazing.

> There are moments where a golden hour might not be possible. If baby was born in a condition where they need extra help – maybe they're having trouble breathing, their oxygen levels are low or they need a bit of resuscitation – they might be taken to a special care area or neonatal unit, but this should be communicated to you, and you should still get a chance to bond as soon as it's safe for both of you.

TRAINING YOUR MIND (WITHOUT THE CRINGE)

Let's get one thing straight – I know this all sounds cheesy. 'Train your mind' sounds like something you'd see on a Pinterest board next to a smoothie bowl, and I am *the first* person to roll my eyes at that sort of thing. But mark my words: *your mindset can genuinely change the birth you have* or, at the very least, *how you feel about the birth you have.* And that perception matters. It shapes how you experience labour, how you recover, how you tell your birth story later. I'm not here to sell you 'good vibes only', I'm here to help you build a mindset that's honest, unshakeable and *real*.

When I talk about mindset, I don't mean pretending everything's fine when it's not. I mean being mentally

THE BIG PUSH (LITERALLY)

prepared for the truth. Contractions? They're probably going to hurt. Birth? It might get messy, loud, slow, fast or not go to plan. But how will *you* deal with it? That's where mindset comes in. This is about training - not tricking - your mind. Let's get into it.

WHAT DOES 'TRAINING YOUR MIND' ACTUALLY LOOK LIKE?

Understanding Pain vs. Suffering

The Truth. Labour pain is purposeful. It's your body *working*. But suffering is what happens when you feel out of control,scared or alone. Pain you can handle. Suffering? That's when you need tools.

What You Can Do

- **Name the pain.** During contractions, don't panic. Try saying: *'This is temporary. This is doing something.'* It helps shift your mindset from 'I'm in danger' to 'I'm progressing.'
- **Create a 'pain playlist'.** A list of phrases you (or your birth partner) can repeat:
  - 'This pain has purpose.'
  - 'Every wave brings my baby closer.'
  - 'My body is working with me, not against me.'
- **Journal your fears.** Write out what's scaring you about birth. Seeing it in black and white helps you deal with it logically instead of emotionally.

> ### TRY THIS: THE ICE BOWL EXERCISE
>
> This one's powerful. I do it with my mamas all the time.
>
> Get a bowl, fill it with cold water and ice. Dip your hand in. Hold it there. Do it twice.
>
> **Round 1:** No music. No affirmations. No support. Just silence. Most people take their hand out quickly. Because discomfort, with no mental support, feels unbearable.
>
> **Round 2:** Play some music you love. Let someone say kind, grounding words to you. Breathe deeply.
>
> *Stay present.* You'll notice you can hold your hand in longer.
>
> This isn't about proving anything. It's about showing you how mindset, encouragement and support completely change how you experience pain.
>
> It teaches:
>
> 1. You can go further with support.
> 2. Pain doesn't always equal panic.
> 3. You're stronger than you think – with the right tools.

Accepting the Unknown

The Truth. Birth will humble you. That beautifully written birth plan? It's a guide, not a guarantee. Plans might shift, and that's okay.

THE BIG PUSH (LITERALLY)

What You Can Do

- **Write a flexible birth plan.** Use open language like *'If possible . . .'* or *'My preference is . . .'*
- Play out 'what if' scenarios:
  - *If you needed a C-section, what would help you feel calm and informed?*
  - *If your water doesn't break, how will you manage expectations?*
- **Create a Plan B (and C).** One version for your ideal birth, and one for if things change. That's not negativity – it's power.

Prepping Your Inner Voice

The Truth. Your inner voice becomes the loudest in the room during labour. If she's critical, you're battling yourself. If she's kind, you'll feel held.

What You Can Do

- **Record yourself.** Say three grounded affirmations in your voice. Play them during early labour.
- **Mirror practice.** Stand in front of the mirror and say:
  - 'I trust my body.'
  - 'I can do this, even when it feels like I can't.'
  - 'I'm doing the work, and it's working.'
- **Watch your daily self-talk.** Every time you catch yourself being negative during pregnancy, flip it. Training starts *now*.

- **Daily breathwork (even just 5 mins).** Inhale 4, hold 4, exhale 6. Practise during pregnancy so it becomes automatic in labour.
- **Pick a grounding object.** A textured item, necklace or something to hold and focus on through contractions.

Visualising the Hard Bits Too

The Truth. Don't just imagine the perfect water birth with candles. Prepare mentally for the tough bits too – and how you'll *handle* them.

What You Can Do
- Visualise real scenarios:
    - A slow dilation.
    - An unexpected intervention.
    - Needing to advocate for yourself. Picture it. Then picture how you *cope*.
- Do 'If This, Then That' planning:
    - *If* I feel overwhelmed → *Then* I breathe, anchor and ask for space.
    - *If* I get discouraged → *Then* my partner reminds me how far I've come.
- **Visualise your recovery too.** Post-birth, what will make you feel proud, even if it wasn't the birth you imagined?
- **Prep your birth partner.** Give them scripts! Don't leave them guessing.

THE BIG PUSH (LITERALLY)

- 'When I look scared, remind me I'm safe.'
- 'Say: "This is temporary. You're doing amazing."'

You don't need to be super zen. You don't need to chant under a full moon (unless that's your thing). But you *do* need to train your mind so when the D-Day comes, you show up with calm, with power and with tools that serve you.

LET'S TALK HYPNOBIRTHING

Okay, let's start with the truth: I used to think hypnobirthing was a bag of absolute bull. The first time I heard about it, I was like, 'Sorry – you're going to *breathe* your baby out?' I couldn't wrap my head around it. To this day, there are still parts that, in my honest opinion, are a bit of a bag of poo. I'm not going to sugar-coat it.

The first time I heard someone say 'surges' instead of 'contractions', I rolled my eyes so hard my vision was blurry for five minutes. I thought, *Just say what it is!* But honestly? Now I'm all for it. *If it works for the woman, it works.* If calling it a surge instead of a contraction helps her stay calm, focused and in control, then I'm here for it.

Some of the strongest, most focused women I have *ever* seen in labour? They practised hypnobirthing. And not in a 'I made a vision board and then panicked through the whole thing' way. I mean properly practised – calm, collected, present, breathing with purpose, in control of their space. That's when I had to take a step back and say: okay. The mind is actually powerful beyond measure.

So let's get into what it really is and what's actually worth taking from it.

WHAT IS HYPNOBIRTHING, REALLY?

At its core, hypnobirthing is about using your *mind* to influence your *body*. It's not hypnosis like the dramatic stuff you see on telly. Nobody's dangling a stopwatch or making you bark like a dog. It's self-hypnosis. A way of calming your nervous system so deeply that your body feels safe enough to do what it was made to do.

It's a toolkit, not a belief system. It's about reducing fear, increasing calm and creating the right environment – mentally, emotionally and physically – for birth to unfold more smoothly. Fear triggers tension. Tension makes pain feel worse. And that fear-tension-pain cycle is what hypnobirthing aims to break. It's about giving your brain a job to do while your body is doing the rest. And the best part? You don't have to believe in *all* of it to benefit from *some* of it.

HYPNOBIRTHING TECHNIQUES THAT ACTUALLY WORK

Here are some of the core techniques used in hypnobirthing that are genuinely worth your time. You can practise these

THE BIG PUSH (LITERALLY)

during pregnancy and then use them during labour and birth – whether you're having a home birth, a hospital birth or something in between.

Breathwork

Up-breathing for contractions (also called 'surges' in hypnobirthing language): Inhale slowly through your nose for four counts, exhale gently through your mouth for six to eight. This slows your heart rate and keeps oxygen flowing to your uterus and baby, which helps both of you stay calm and steady.

And here's the thing: it's *completely okay* to change the rhythm if that particular count doesn't feel right. The goal is not perfection – it's *presence*. Keep your breathing regulated and unrushed. Sometimes, if you're listening to hypnobirthing audio, the pace might not match where *you're* at. It might feel too fast, too slow or just not quite right, and that's okay. You don't need to stick to a script. Go with your own body's rhythm. As long as your breathing is steady and intentional, you're doing it right.

Why this works: Your breath is your control centre. The deeper and calmer your breathing, the more your body believes it's safe. And a body that feels safe opens more easily.

Affirmations

These are positive, empowering statements that you repeat regularly. They rewire your internal dialogue and become your go-to script when things get intense. Examples:

- 'My body was made for this.'
- 'I'm calm. I'm safe. I'm strong.'
- 'Each wave brings my baby closer.'

Why this works: Your brain absorbs language. When you feed it calm, supportive words during pregnancy, those are the words it reaches for in labour, especially when you feel like you're losing control. You can record affirmations in your own voice, listen to guided ones online, or write your own that feel true to *you*. The more personalised, the better.

Visualisation

This means using your imagination to picture something calming and empowering. It could be:

- Your cervix opening like a blooming flower.
- A wave rising, peaking and falling – matching your contraction.
- A calm, peaceful room with you holding your baby afterwards.

Why this works: Your brain doesn't know the difference between real calm and imagined calm. If you've visualised yourself handling tough moments, you're more likely to stay calm *in* them.

Touch and Anchoring

This involves using consistent touch or a cue word to bring yourself back to calm. For example, during pregnancy, you might practise having your birth partner gently press on your shoulder or rub your lower back while you breathe. Pair this touch with a calming word or phrase. Eventually, your body associates that touch with relaxation. Then, in labour, that same touch can help trigger a calming response without you even thinking.

Why this works: It gives your brain a shortcut. When your birth partner does the thing you've practised, your body goes, 'Ah - we're okay.' The body remembers. All we're doing here is training your brain to respond to a specific cue with calm instead of chaos.

Controlling Your Environment

Hypnobirthing places big importance on the environment. That's because mammals give birth best in warm, private, familiar spaces. So you want to make your birth space feel as calm and comfortable as possible. That might mean:

- Dimming the lights.
- Playing calming music or nature sounds.
- Using essential oils or familiar scents.
- Limiting unnecessary interruptions.

Why this works: Your brain associates certain conditions with safety. The more calm and private you feel, the more your body can let go.

HYPNOBIRTHING AND FAITH – CAN THEY COEXIST?

Let's just address the elephant in the room. For some of you, the word *hypnobirthing* already has you clutching your Bible, your Quran or side-eyeing this whole section like, *'Sis, is this not witchcraft?'* I've heard it all – 'It sounds demonic,' 'Isn't that a spiritual ritual?', 'They're in a cult.' And honestly? I get it.

When you've grown up in a faith-filled environment, anything that sounds even slightly mystical or unfamiliar can trigger discomfort. I felt the same way at first. The name alone had me squinting. And I won't lie, there are definitely elements of hypnobirthing out there that didn't (and still don't) sit right with me.

Here's what I've learned over the years: you can take what works for you and leave what doesn't. At its core, hypnobirthing is simply about calming the mind and giving the body a safer, more relaxed space to do its work. It's about learning to control your breath, stay grounded in intense moments and feel empowered through the process, emotionally and physically.

THE BIG PUSH (LITERALLY)

You're not being asked to replace your beliefs or follow any new philosophy. In fact, you can bring your faith into it. Many people I've supported have done this beautifully. They've prayed between contractions. They've listened to gospel, nasheeds or worship music while breathing through surges. They've used scripture as affirmations. There are even faith-based hypnobirthing resources available – affirmations and audio tracks rooted in biblical truths or other spiritual foundations. Things like:

- 'God is with me through every surge.'
- 'I am fearfully and wonderfully made.'
- 'I can do all things through Christ who strengthens me.'

You can speak the name of God while using every tool in this book. You can centre yourself in your faith and still benefit from breathing techniques and visualisations. None of it has to be in conflict. If certain words or phrases don't align with your beliefs, you are completely free to switch them out for ones that do. This is your birth, your journey, your truth. If your first instinct was 'this isn't for me,' I understand. But just know: you're still welcome here. You can engage with these techniques through the lens of your own faith and values. You get to choose what serves you and what doesn't.

HOW TO PUSH (AND WHY THE INTERNET ISN'T ALWAYS RIGHT)

Let's talk about how to push. I've seen so much stuff online that genuinely irritates my soul. A part of me just wants to scream, *Stop lying to women.* There is so much information floating around, and while some of it is well-meaning, a lot of it is misleading or at best, only half the story.

One common line I keep seeing is: *You don't need to push. Your body does it for you.* The idea comes from a good place: trusting your body, tuning in – and there's *some* truth to it. Your body **can** push your baby out without conscious effort (the **foetal ejection reflex**), but here's the issue: when people throw around these phrases without the full science, without the full reality of birth, it can be incredibly damaging. Women cling to what they hear, especially in a world where we're desperate for answers and reassurance. If you're going to give advice, give the full truth – not a filtered Instagram-caption version.

THE FOETAL EJECTION REFLEX: MAGICAL, BUT NOT GUARANTEED

Your body *can* push the baby out on its own without you doing anything. That's the foetal ejection reflex. It's powerful, involuntary and often happens when you feel completely safe, unobserved and undisturbed – usually without pain

THE BIG PUSH (LITERALLY)

medication, and more commonly if it's not your first birth. When it happens, it's incredible. Your uterus contracts, your baby descends and you might literally feel your body take over, doing exactly what it was designed to do.

But let me tell you now: **not everyone experiences this**. Pretending like it's the standard experience is unfair. If *everyone* could just 'breathe their baby out', we'd have babies sliding out on yoga mats left and right. But for a lot of women, labour is intense. Pushing is hard. It takes *effort*, and that doesn't mean something's gone wrong – it means you're human.

SO, HOW SHOULD YOU PUSH?

Traditionally – and in every class I've ever taught – I tell women: **'Push like you're doing a poo.'** It's clear, it activates the right muscles, and it gives women a sense of control. You tuck your chin, take a deep breath in, bear down into your bum, and push with intention. You're focusing your power where it needs to go. I've watched that method bring babies into this world safely and efficiently time and time again.

But recently, some research has suggested that this type of straining, especially over long periods, might increase your risk of haemorrhoids or worsen existing ones. Studies have shown that prolonged closed-glottis pushing (holding your breath and bearing down hard) may put excess pressure on the pelvic floor and rectal area. So it's worth considering the impact. That's why I now say this: **pushing like you're doing a poo can absolutely work, but it's not the only way.** If you find yourself pushing for ages and feeling like nothing's happening, or you're just getting more and more exhausted, it's okay to pause. Re-centre. Try something else.

Here are some alternatives you can use, or combine with the 'poo push', depending on how you're feeling and what your body is doing.

- **Open-Glottis Pushing.** Instead of holding your breath and bearing down, breathe out slowly while pushing. It reduces pressure and may lessen your risk of perineal trauma.
- **Spontaneous Pushing.** Wait for the natural urge. Let your body tell you when to push and just follow it.
- **Upright Positions.** Kneeling, squatting or using a birth stool can let gravity help. You may find you need less effort to push.
- **Perineal Support.** Some midwives apply warm compresses or gentle massage to help reduce tearing and improve stretch.

HOW LONG DOES PUSHING LAST? (SPOILER: IT VARIES)

Let's talk about how long pushing can actually take. I've seen it all. From women who didn't even make it out of the lift before their baby arrived, to those who pushed for two,

THE BIG PUSH (LITERALLY)

even two and a half hours. The truth is, the length of the pushing stage varies widely and depends on several factors, including whether it's your first baby, the baby's position, and whether you've had an epidural.

What the Research Says

- **First-time mothers.** Pushing can last up to **three hours**, especially if an epidural is used.
- **Mothers who've given birth before.** Pushing typically lasts up to **two hours**.

These are general guidelines. For some, it'll be shorter. For others, longer. And every scenario is valid.

WHAT CAN HELP REDUCE PUSHING TIME?

If you're 10cm dilated and both you and your baby are doing well, one really helpful thing to consider is **not starting to push straight away**. Just because you're fully dilated doesn't mean you need to jump into action. If your baby's head is still quite high, your team might suggest that you **mobilise**: walk around the room, do some gentle squats, or use a birthing ball. This is called **'labouring down'**. It gives your baby time to descend naturally into the pelvis, which can lead to:

- Shorter pushing time.
- Less exhaustion for you.
- More effective pushing when the time comes.

Even if you've had an epidural and you can't walk around, all is not lost. There are still **positions** you can try in bed that can help your baby move down and rotate into the best position for birth:

- Side-lying with a peanut ball between your knees.
- Hands and knees (if you've got enough movement).
- Semi-reclined with knees wide.
- Lunging or kneeling using the bed for support.

Using gravity, hip-opening positions and space for baby to move can be game-changing.

So if you're fully dilated and not yet feeling that overwhelming urge to push, and both of you are well, **it's okay to pause**. Use that time to breathe, to move (if you can) and to let baby come down a little more on their own. It might save you energy later when you need it most.

If baby's really stressed, or if you're really tired or if your temperature's rising and there's a risk of infection, your healthcare team might decide it's time to get baby out more quickly. That could mean encouraging pushing even if the head's not as low, or using instruments to assist.

But the key takeaway is this: **pushing can take minutes or it can take hours – it's not one-size-fits-all**. It depends on the baby, your body, your birth plan and what's safest in that moment. Trust your team. Trust your body. And know that if it takes a while, that's okay.

THE BIG PUSH (LITERALLY)

TEARS, BUT NOT THE EMOTIONAL KIND

I would love to conduct a survey to ask what women are most scared of when it comes to labour, and I can bet my little-to-no savings that it's tearing. Women fear tearing more than caesareans. If I could come up with a product that meant women would never tear again, I'd start looking for my mansion in the Bahamas because me and my unborn kids would never have to work again. While I don't have that idea just yet, let's discuss tearing.

The perineum is the space between your vagina and your anus. Don't be shy – you should squat over a mirror and have a look and know what your anatomy looks like. Essentially, its role is to support your pelvic floor muscles and maintain continence, which is a fancy way of saying you can control when you wee and poo. Perineal tears are common. Let's state the obvious: it's not every Thursday that a whole human comes out of your vagina, so give yourself grace. Over 70 per cent of women who have a vaginal birth will experience some type of perineal tear. Tears come in different categories.

- **A first-degree tear** is like a graze, a second-degree tear is like a cut. These tears are the most common. Most times, we leave a first-degree tear alone

because they're tiny and we'd probably cause more trauma trying to suture them together.
- **Second-degree tears** are the most common, with the majority requiring suturing. Both first- and second-degree tears can be sutured by a midwife. These tears are our bread and butter – we see them all the time.
- **A third-degree tear** means it's hit muscle. Midwives don't do muscles – we are fragile peeps. Doctors have to suture third- and fourth degree tears, and this requires strong anaesthesia, such as a spinal, which is an injection in the lower back that numbs you from the waist down.
- **Fourth-degree tears** are rare, and I'm lucky to say that in my six years of being a midwife, I have never seen one. A fourth-degree tear is when a woman tears all the way to her bum hole. As I'm typing, I'm even crossing my legs. This is rare. I repeat, this is rare, and no, don't start thinking it'd be just your luck to have a fourth-degree tear – get it out of your mind.

The best mindset to have going into labour is this: *I'm aiming for no tear, but if I do tear, I hope it's small and easily sutured.* Preparation is key. Yes, perineal tears are common, but there are things you can do to lower the chances and reduce the severity. Now, outside of perineal tears, there are actually six other types of tears. Please don't panic – I slipped that fact into this paragraph on purpose. I won't go into too much detail about them because they're not as common.

THE BIG PUSH (LITERALLY)

Take vaginal tears, for example – there's nothing you can do to prevent them, so there's no point in stressing over them.

Now, let's focus on the good stuff – how to reduce the extent of a tear.

PERINEAL MASSAGE: TRAINING FOR THE BIG DAY

Now, there are mixed messages about this, with some saying it's nonsense and some swearing by it, so let's start with what research says.

Does perineal massage actually help? Yep, science says it does. Regularly massaging the perineum in late pregnancy has been shown to reduce the chances of severe tearing – those dreaded third- and fourth-degree ones that go deep into the muscle and anal sphincter. It also lowers the likelihood of needing an episiotomy, which is when a small cut is made to widen the vaginal opening during birth. And the best part? Women who practised perineal massage reported less pain in the months after giving birth. Giving your perineum a little TLC before labour can make birth easier and postpartum recovery smoother. Worth a shot, right?

Now, I'm an honest babe. I've looked at a lot of research on perineal massage. Yes, studies show it helps, but the numbers aren't groundbreaking. That said, I'm a big believer in: *if it won't harm you and there's even a small chance it could help, why not give it a go?* Most experts recommend starting around 34 to 36 weeks of pregnancy and continuing

2-3 times a week until birth. Some women prefer to do it daily, but even once or twice a week can make a difference. It's best to do it after a warm bath or shower when the tissues are softer and more elastic.

When I think of perineal massage, I picture going to the gym. If I tried to bench press on my first day, I wouldn't jump straight to heavy weights - I'd start with just the bar, then add 5kg, then 10kg, and gradually build up strength. Now, apply that same logic to your perineum. Your perineum is a muscle, and your baby? Well, that's a 30kg weight. What you *don't* want is for the first time your perineum stretches to be when your baby's head is crowning. Massage it, get it used to the stretch, and *hopefully*, you won't tear. And remember - if you do, the goal is to keep it as minimal as possible.

THE POWER OF A WARM COMPRESS: SMALL ACTION, BIG IMPACT

Let's talk about warming up, because it's just as important when it comes to birth. Midwives and researchers have found that applying a warm, damp cloth to the perineum while pushing can reduce the risk of severe tears and make things a little more comfortable. Studies show that women who use warm compresses during birth are *less likely* to experience third- and fourth-degree tears.

So what's the science behind a warm compress? Heat increases blood flow, making the tissues more flexible and better able to stretch rather than tear. It's the same reason

THE BIG PUSH (LITERALLY)

you warm up before a workout – your muscles and skin become more pliable. On top of that, the gentle pressure from the compress supports the perineum, slows things down, and helps your body adjust as the baby's head crowns. Basically, the warm compress and pressure are having a heart-to-heart with your perineum, saying: 'Babe, you've got this.' Midwives are trained to do this, but don't assume it'll just happen. Put it in your birth plan, and make sure your birth partner reminds the midwife when the time comes.

CONTROLLED PUSHING: THE RING OF FIRE VS. THE RED SEA

Another way to lower your chances of tearing is by controlling how you push. Think *gentle*, not launching your baby into the world like a rocket. As your baby's head starts to emerge, you'll experience what many call the *ring of fire.* This is when the widest part of your baby's head is stretching your perineum. Now, this is where technique matters. I tell all my mums to imagine they're blowing out candles when it gets to that moment. Your instinct might be to *push hard* to get it over with, but try your best not to. The ring of fire hurts for a moment, but parting like the Red Sea? That pain lasts a lot longer. And yes, I'm still crossing my legs.

Let's go over this: you're pushing, pushing, pushing, baby is coming, your midwife suddenly says *stop!* This is your cue to switch to candle mode. Picture a cake with 12 candles all around it. Blow them out one by one. Then, when your midwife gives the green light, do *small, controlled pushes* until your baby's head is delivered. Remember: don't *spit* baby out. Breathe, blow your candles and *hopefully* you won't tear, and if you do, it'll be minimal.

PUSH SMARTER, NOT HARDER: THE BEST BIRTH POSITIONS FOR YOUR PERINEUM

I hate cancel culture, but if there's one thing I *fully* support cancelling, it's encouraging everyone to give birth lying flat with your legs up. Not only is this position outdated, but it also increases the risk of tearing by reducing space in the pelvis and putting extra pressure on the perineum. And honestly? That's just plain evil – the babe is already going through enough! Instead, positions like side-lying, hands-and-knees, squatting or kneeling allow the perineum to stretch more gradually, easing the strain. Research even shows that side-lying significantly lowers the risk of severe tears. So if you want to be kinder to your perineum, explore different positions when pushing – you've got options!

VAGINAL EXAMINATIONS: THE TRUTH, THE PURPOSE AND THE POWER ARE STILL YOURS

I know just saying the words makes some people feel instantly tense. For some, the thought of a care provider

THE BIG PUSH (LITERALLY)

putting fingers inside you during labour sounds invasive, scary, unnecessary and even traumatic. Vaginal examinations can be uncomfortable. They can feel intimate, clinical or just plain annoying.

There's a lot of online talk right now about how they're not needed, and how 'you should just let your body do what it needs to do', and yes, that's true in some cases. You can absolutely go through your entire labour without a single vaginal examination. And if that's your choice, that's valid. But let's also keep it real: **sometimes, a vaginal examination gives us key information that shapes your care plan in a big way**. It's not just about 'how many centimetres dilated you are'. It's about getting a full picture of what's going on.

WHAT IS A VAGINAL EXAMINATION ACTUALLY FOR?

When a care provider does a vaginal examination, they are checking for a *lot* more than just dilation. Here's what they're looking for:

- **How open your cervix is** (measured in centimetres, usually up to 10cm for full dilation).
- **The consistency of the cervix** – is it soft, stretchy or still firm?
- **The position of the cervix** – anterior, posterior, central?
- **How far down the baby's head is** – also known as baby's *station*.

- What direction baby is facing – back-to-back or well positioned?
- How engaged the head is in the pelvis.

So when you hear someone say, 'You're 4cm,' that number is only part of the story. Someone can be 4cm with a thick cervix and baby still floating high, or 4cm with a paper-thin cervix and baby nearly on the doorstep. It's not about numbers – it's about the *whole picture.*

WHEN MIGHT VAGINAL EXAMINATIONS BE OFFERED?

If you're in established labour, care providers may offer vaginal examinations every **four to six hours**. The aim is to see whether labour is progressing safely and whether your body is responding well to the contractions. Sometimes care providers get a little too eager, constantly suggesting another exam – and that can be tiring. **Your vagina is not a 'what's-in-the-box' prize.** You don't have to be checked just for the sake of it.

That said, there *are* moments when a vaginal examination is incredibly useful and important:

- If your baby's heart rate drops and your care team needs to decide whether to assist the birth or move to a caesarean.
- If you're having regular contractions but progress seems to have stalled.

THE BIG PUSH (LITERALLY)

- If you're being induced and your provider needs to assess whether your cervix is favourable, or what method would work best.
- If you've been pushing for a long time and they want to check baby's position.
- If you're approaching 41–42 weeks and your team is considering induction, a vaginal exam might help decide what kind of induction would be most suitable.

Equally, there are times when vaginal examinations might not be advised at all:

- If your **waters have broken**, especially if they've been broken for a while – we don't want to increase the risk of infection.
- If you're **not in active labour yet,** and we're trying not to over-intervene.
- If you're **premature,** because touching the cervix could stimulate labour too early.
- Or simply – if you don't want one, and there's no clinical reason to do it.

IT'S OKAY TO SAY NO AND IT'S OKAY TO SAY YES

This part is so important: **you can decline a vaginal examination at any time.** Even if a care provider offers one, even if they're wearing gloves and ready to go, you are *never* obligated to say yes. You can say:

- 'No, not right now.'
- 'Can we wait another hour?'
- 'I'd like to talk about why this is necessary.'

Let me also say this: **it's okay to say yes, too**. Some women feel reassured knowing how far along they are. Some want to understand what's happening in their body. Some just want a sense of where things are at. That is just as valid. This is your birth. You're allowed to want the information, and you're allowed to protect your space. Both things can exist at the same time.

MAKING IT MORE COMFORTABLE

Vaginal examinations can be painful or just really uncomfortable, especially during contractions. But there are ways to make the process gentler and your care provider should support you through every step.

Here's what should happen:

- They should explain exactly what they're going to do *before* they do it.

THE BIG PUSH (LITERALLY)

- They should show you that the gel is cold (when I examine, I do this by putting a bit of the gel on mum's vulva to show her it's cold so she knows what sensation is coming).
- They should ask for your consent *every single time*.
- They should talk you through the process gently and clearly.
- You should feel **in control** – you can ask them to slow down, talk more, stop at any point.
- And if at any time you feel overwhelmed or unsafe, **you can say 'stop', and they must stop.**

You can also use your breath to relax your body – deep, slow inhales and long exhales. You might ask your birth partner to hold your hand or place a calming hand on your shoulder or back. You can also ask for silence, music or whatever helps you ground yourself.

The bottom line is that information is power, but the power is still yours. Vaginal examinations are a **tool**. They can be helpful, they can be necessary, and sometimes, they're not needed at all. You are the one giving birth. **You decide what you're comfortable with.** So whether you go your entire labour without a single examination, ask for one when you feel ready, or request them regularly to stay informed – you are allowed to choose. And whatever you choose, you deserve to feel safe, respected and fully in control.

STUDENT MIDWIVES: SHOULD YOU HAVE ONE IN THE ROOM?

I *love* student midwives. I can't even pretend otherwise. Because I was one, and let me tell you, I fought for my life during every single shift. I get it, though. It's your big day, your birth. You want the best of the best. You might feel a bit iffy when you're asked, *'Would you mind if a student midwife is present?'* because in your mind, this isn't a training session, this is *your* moment. And you're absolutely right – it is. But I want to shift your perspective a little.

Student midwives aren't there to 'experiment' on you. They're there to **learn,** and they learn under the supervision of qualified midwives at all times.* These students are going to qualify anyway. Very soon, they'll be leading care themselves. So the more hands-on, real experience they get now, the better, safer and more confident they'll be when it really is just them in that room. If I'm being completely honest, there wasn't much of a difference between the shifts I did as a final-year student and the day after I qualified when the system said, 'Congrats – you're on your own.'

Student midwives are often the ones with the most up-to-date, evidence-based knowledge. You'd be surprised how

---

* Well . . . most times. I won't lie: once, my supervising midwife popped out for a cup of tea and before she came back, the baby's head was out. But hey – baby was fine, mum was fine, and here I am today, still standing!

THE BIG PUSH (LITERALLY)

many times even qualified midwives (me included) have been gently corrected by a student. Not because we didn't know our stuff, but because things change so fast. When you're knee-deep working on the wards, you're so busy documenting, caring, managing emergencies, that you don't always have time to read the newest research articles. Students, fresh from lectures and placements, are often the ones bringing the latest evidence into the room. They're a walking, talking, human update, and that is something to be respected.

As a midwife, you also work better when you have a student midwife by your side. You've got another pair of eyes. Another voice in the room. Another advocate standing with you, and for you. Some of the best care I ever gave was when I was a student.

Students are often the ones noticing that your water bottle's empty, that your hair needs tying back, that your partner needs a chair. They're the ones offering that gentle hand rub, wiping your brow, quietly advocating for your wishes when the room gets busy and overwhelming. While the midwife has to be focused on monitoring and documenting (because trust me, the paperwork load is real), the student often has that little bit more breathing space to really see you, to pick up the little things, to make you feel human in a moment that can otherwise start to feel a bit clinical.

If you've got this far in this book, you know that I tell the truth and the whole truth. I understand why some women can be scared about having a student midwife in the room. You're scared yourself and you feel like there's now another person who does not know what they're doing, and I totally get that. I also want to give you some practical reassurance. For example, if you're worried about a student doing a vaginal examination, you can absolutely ask for the midwife to do it first. In fact, that's even better because if the midwife's examination is really uncomfortable or doesn't feel right, you can say no straight away, without worrying about the student's feelings. If the midwife goes first, you have more control and more confidence to say no if you need to. And if you do say yes, the midwife can directly supervise the student and guide their hands.

You get to decide what's comfortable for you. If you feel like having a student there would add too much stress, that's okay, but you'd be surprised at how amazing they can be and how comforting it can feel to have them there. Plus, remember: student midwives have to do observation births, so if they're supporting you, you're probably not the first, and if you were the first, they wouldn't be doing anything hands-on. My own student midwives watch a few births first, then they put their hands on top of mine so they can learn what I'm feeling, and only after that do they do anything on their own.

Your birth. Your rules. Always. No one should ever make you feel bad for saying no. But if you're able, if you feel safe, if your gut says yes, give a student midwife a chance. You might be surprised at how much you get back in return. You won't just be helping them - you'll often be getting some of the most heartfelt, attentive care there is.

If you've had a bad experience with a student midwife before, I hear you. I really do. But remember, one bad experience doesn't mean they're all the same. It's the same way that one bad experience with a midwife wouldn't mean you should now plan a freebirth alone in your bathroom. Student midwives are the future. They are the hands that will one day catch babies, wipe tears, advocate fiercely and walk people through the best, and sometimes the hardest, days of their lives.

WHEN THINGS DON'T GO TO PLAN

Labour is such a moment of precision - every contraction, every movement, every heartbeat matters. But with anything that requires precision, there's always room for things to go slightly off course. Emergencies in labour aren't exactly rare, and while that might sound scary, what it really means is that your team is very experienced in recognising and handling them quickly.

Some of the more common emergencies include:

- **Shoulder dystocia** – when the baby's shoulder gets stuck after the head is born. One of the first things we try is changing your position – having you get on your hands and knees or pull your knees right up to your chest, which we call the **McRoberts manoeuvre**.

These simple movements can create more space in your pelvis and often help the baby's shoulder slip free. In more complex cases, a midwife or doctor might use what we call a **Pringle hand**, gently placing a hand inside the vagina in a scooping motion, a bit like reaching for the last Pringle in the tube, to help release the shoulder safely.

- **Postpartum haemorrhage (PPH)** – heavy bleeding after birth, treated quickly with medication, fluids, or other interventions to control it.
- **Foetal bradycardia** – when the baby's heart rate drops and doesn't recover, which may lead to an assisted or caesarean birth.
- **Undiagnosed breech** – when a baby is unexpectedly bottom- or foot-first in labour, sometimes requiring a change in delivery plan.
- **Pre-eclampsia and eclampsia** – linked to high blood pressure and can cause headaches, swelling or seizures if untreated.
- **Cord prolapse** – when the umbilical cord slips down before the baby, reducing oxygen flow and needing immediate attention.

These situations sound intense, but every midwife and doctor in that room has practised these responses over and over again. The point isn't to make you anxious, it's to remind you that birth is both powerful and unpredictable, and you'll be surrounded by people who know exactly what to do.

THE BIG PUSH (LITERALLY)

DIFFERENT WAYS TO MEET YOUR BABY

Because every journey is a celebration - we're just choosing the venue.

When you picture giving birth, you might have a specific scene in your mind. Maybe a spontaneous vaginal delivery where everything flows smoothly, maybe a planned caesarean, or maybe something in between. The truth is, there are several different ways babies make their grand entrance into the world, and all of them are valid. In this chapter, we're going to break down the three main types of birth: spontaneous vaginal birth, assisted vaginal birth (using instruments like forceps or ventouse) and C-section (both elective and emergency). We'll talk about what each birth entails, why it might happen, what recovery can look like, and most importantly, why how your baby is born does not determine how strong you are.

VAGINAL BIRTH (SPONTANEOUS VAGINAL DELIVERY)

What It Is: A spontaneous vaginal birth is when labour starts naturally or is gently encouraged (like with an induction), and the baby is born through the birth canal without the need for instruments or surgery.

I'M PREGNANT ... NOW WHAT?

Why It's Often Preferred (When Safe)
- **Quicker Recovery:** Vaginal births typically come with the shortest physical recovery time compared to assisted or caesarean births.
- **Lower Risks:** There's no surgical wound to heal, and the risks of blood clots, infections and other surgical complications are lower.
- **Shorter Hospital Stay:** Many women are able to go home within six–24 hours after an uncomplicated vaginal birth.
- **Bonding and Breastfeeding:** Early skin-to-skin and breastfeeding can often happen immediately (though of course, it can with caesareans too – with a little adjustment).

When It's Ideal
- Pregnancy has been low-risk throughout.
- Baby is in a head-down (vertex) position.
- Labour is progressing well and safely for both mother and baby.

Recovery
- Expect some vaginal bleeding (lochia) for up to six weeks.
- Soreness around the perineum, especially if there are minor tears or grazes.
- Practise pelvic floor exercises – they are essential even if you didn't have a tear! (If you're not sure how

THE BIG PUSH (LITERALLY)

to do them, ask your midwife, physiotherapist, or check one of the trusted resources listed at the back of this book.)
- Emotional recovery is just as important – some vaginal births can feel fast and overwhelming, while others feel slow and exhausting. There's no right or wrong.

INSTRUMENTAL OR ASSISTED VAGINAL BIRTH

What It Is: An instrumental or assisted birth uses tools - either **forceps** (think of big metal tongs) or a **ventouse** (a suction cap) - to help deliver the baby vaginally.

Why Might We Need It?
- **Baby's Safety:** If the baby's heart rate shows signs of distress and needs to be born quickly.
- **Maternal Exhaustion:** Labour can be long and draining; sometimes a mum just doesn't have the energy to push any more – and that's okay.
- **Medical Concerns:** Conditions like **maternal sepsis, pre-eclampsia** or heavy bleeding can mean speeding up the birth is safer.
- **Failure to Progress:** If labour stalls at the very end (for example, pushing for a long time without progress), an instrument may help complete the journey.

I'M PREGNANT ... NOW WHAT?

What It Could Involve

- Sometimes an **episiotomy** (a small cut to widen the vaginal opening) is needed to help the instruments work safely.
- Swelling or bruising around the baby's head is common (especially with ventouse), but usually resolves quickly.
- You might feel tender around the perineum and pelvic floor.

Recovery

- Can involve a bit more soreness than a straightforward vaginal birth.
- Healing of any stitches (whether from tears or episiotomy) is crucial.
- Emotional recovery is important too – some women feel surprised or upset by needing assistance, even when it was the safest choice.

Important Reminder: Needing help doesn't make your birth any less 'natural' or any less yours. **You birthed your baby.** You just had a little help when it was needed most.

CAESAREAN SECTION BIRTH

What It Is: A caesarean section (or C-section) is major surgery where your baby is delivered through an incision made in your abdomen and womb. There are two broad types: **elective** and **emergency** caesareans.

Elective (Planned) Caesarean

What It Is: A planned C-section booked ahead of time, usually between 38–39 weeks, before you go into labour.

Why You Might Have One
- **Breech Baby**: Especially a footling breech where feet are positioned to come out first – considered too risky for vaginal birth.
- **Twins or Multiples:** Particularly if babies are lying sideways (transverse) or if Twin 1 (the first one to come out) isn't head-down.
- **Placenta Praevia:** Where the placenta is covering the cervix, making vaginal birth dangerous.
- **Previous Birth Complications:** Such as a third- or fourth-degree tear.
- **Maternal Health Concerns**: Heart conditions, severe pre-eclampsia, etc.
- **Maternal Request:** Some women choose an elective caesarean for personal, psychological or physical reasons after being counselled on risks and benefits.

Important Note: An elective caesarean is still a birth – it's still a moment where you meet your baby for the first time. The route might be different, but the destination is just as beautiful.

Emergency Caesarean

What It Is: A C-section decided before or during labour because it becomes safer for mother and/or baby.

Categories of Emergency Caesarean
- **Category 1:** Immediate danger to life – need to deliver within 30 minutes (examples: **cord prolapse, uterine rupture**).
- **Category 2:** Urgent but not immediately life-threatening (example: concerning foetal heart rate, labour not progressing).
- **Category 3:** No immediate risk but need to deliver earlier than planned (example: early labour when a caesarean was already booked for other reasons).

Common Reasons
- Labour not progressing (failure to dilate or descend).
- Signs of foetal distress (heart rate concerns).
- Maternal complications like infection or severe bleeding.

Recovery From Caesarean Birth
Physical Healing:
- Six to eight weeks minimum for abdominal muscles and scar tissue healing.

Hospital Stay:
- Typically two to four days.

THE BIG PUSH (LITERALLY)

Movement:
- Gentle walking as soon as you can to prevent blood clots.

Pain Management:
- Regular pain relief is important – don't try to 'tough it out'.

Emotional Healing:
- It's normal to grieve the birth you hoped for while celebrating the baby you have. Birth can be joyful and disappointing at the same time – you're allowed to feel all of it. And always remember: 'It's still your baby's birthday. Just at a different venue.'

Next Pregnancy Advice:
- Ideally, wait **12–18 months** before trying to conceive again. This gives your womb (especially the scar tissue) the best chance to heal fully and lowers the risk of scar rupture.

FINAL THOUGHTS

Whether your birth is spontaneous, assisted or surgical, **it's still a birth**. It's a profound transformation – the day you become a mother in a whole new way. No matter what path your baby takes to get to you, **you carried them; you nurtured them; you birthed them**. That's what matters most.

MONITORING IN LABOUR: WHAT'S NORMAL, WHAT'S IMPORTANT

During labour, your body and your baby are working together in a powerful dance. To make sure everything is going smoothly, midwives and doctors will keep a close eye on a few key metrics – both yours and baby's. Before labour starts, you might have a baseline blood test to check your iron levels, platelets and other general markers of health. This gives us a picture of what's normal for you, so if anything changes during labour, we can spot it early.

Once labour is underway, we regularly assess:

- **Your blood pressure and pulse** – to make sure your heart is coping well and to check for any signs of pre-eclampsia or infection.
- **Your temperature** – a raised temperature can be an early sign of infection.
- **Your breathing rate** – helps us see if you're getting tired or need extra support.
- **Your baby's heartbeat** – this is a big one, and we have two main ways of listening.

MONITORING BABY'S HEARTBEAT

We listen to baby in two main ways:

THE BIG PUSH (LITERALLY)

1. Intermittent Auscultation (IA)

This is done with a handheld Doppler or a traditional Pinard stethoscope. Every 15 minutes or so in the active first stage of labour, and after every contraction in the second stage, we'll listen to baby's heartbeat for about a minute.

When it's used:

- When your pregnancy has been straightforward and there are no current concerns.
- When everything's progressing normally.
- When you're moving around freely and want to keep things feeling less medicalised.

Why I recommend it: If there are no specific concerns, I always encourage intermittent auscultation. It's safe, supports your movement and comfort and helps keep birth feeling like your own space.

2. Continuous Electronic Foetal Monitoring (CTG)

This involves two sensors strapped around your belly – one to pick up baby's heartbeat and another to monitor your contractions. It continuously traces baby's heart rate and your contractions on paper or a screen.

When it's used:

- If there's a reason to monitor more closely during labour.
- If baby or you need extra reassurance.

- If you're being induced or have an epidural.
- If there are any signs that baby might need a bit more support.

What you might notice: You'll see baby's heart rate patterns, with rises and falls that often reflect their natural sleep and activity cycles. Yes, babies nap, even during labour!

Wireless CTG: Many hospitals now have wireless CTG monitors, which let you move around more freely, even getting into the shower or bath if you like. If you're recommended to have continuous monitoring, ask your hospital if they have wireless CTG available. Staying mobile can help you feel more in control and can really make a difference to how you experience labour.

WHY MONITORING MATTERS

Monitoring is there to pick up any early signs of stress or infection in you or baby. It should always be balanced with your comfort and your choices. The more you can move and the more upright and forward-leaning you can be, the more you can work with your body's natural power. I always say, 'Vagina should face the floor – let gravity help you!'

THE BIG PUSH (LITERALLY)

PAIN RELIEF

PARACETAMOL AND DIHYDROCODEINE (AKA: THE MILD WARRIORS)

Let's be real: **paracetamol on its own doesn't do much in labour**. It doesn't even take away my headache or my period pain now, let alone contractions. But when you pair it with **dihydrocodeine**, it's got a bit more kick. It's usually offered in **early labour** and can take the edge off a bit.

This is what we call **first-tier pain relief**. It's the starting point for most hospitals, and it's typically given in **tablet form**. Different hospitals might use slightly different meds depending on where you are (especially if you're outside the UK), but the concept is the same – it's the **first** stage of medication before you move on to the heavier hitters like **pethidine** or **epidurals**.

And here's something people don't realise: You can **go into hospital, get pain relief, and go back home**. You don't have to stay. This is called **home on analgesia** and it's a great option for early labour babes who aren't quite ready for full admission but want something in their system.

GAS AND AIR: THE ONE YOU CAN KEEP GOING BACK TO

Gas and air is one of the only pain reliefs you can use **as much as you like**. It doesn't affect your baby at all, doesn't stay in your system, and you're in control. Use it properly, though:

- Breathe *in* through the mouthpiece.
- Breathe *out* into the mouthpiece.

You're not smoking shisha. Don't breathe it out into the room. Also, start using it **before the contraction peaks**. If you wait till the pain is fully there, you've missed your moment. It also helps regulate your breathing, something many people don't realise is *pain relief in itself.*

PS. Yes – we all know your partner tries it when we leave the room. Don't worry, we see you.

Let's talk nausea. Some women find that gas and air makes them feel a bit queasy, or even makes them vomit. If that happens, my tip would be:

- Take a break.
- Have a sip of water.
- Then try again, because you've had that first hit of nausea and your body is getting used to it.

And if it's still not sitting right? Ask for **anti-sickness meds**, which can make a huge difference. However, if you find it's just *not your vibe*, if it's making you feel too disconnected or you want to stay fully present in your birth – **that's okay too.** Put it down, breathe through and keep moving. Trust yourself. If you just want to **rule it out** completely

THE BIG PUSH (LITERALLY)

because you prefer to feel **every** moment and stay super present, that's your choice too. You're not missing out on a prize for how many tools you used. Do what feels right.

PETHIDINE: MY UNDERRATED QUEEN

I **love** pethidine. I've seen women go from crying and tensing up to literally melting into the bed within minutes. It won't completely remove the pain, but it **softens** the intensity. That 'I'm about to lose it' bit? Pethidine takes the edge off that.

Here's the science: adrenaline blocks oxytocin and **oxytocin** is what you need for labour to move. When pethidine helps you relax, your body can finally get back to doing what it needs to do.

Why Some Hospitals Don't Use It: The reason some hospitals **don't** offer pethidine, or have started phasing it out, is because it's a medicine that crosses the placenta. It makes **mum** drowsy, and it can make **baby** drowsy too. And if baby comes out a bit too sleepy, they might need some help getting their breathing started, or it might delay their first feed.

When We Don't Give It: Pethidine isn't for everyone. I wouldn't offer it if:

- You're **close to delivery** (because of the placenta crossover, it can make baby too sleepy).
- Baby's **heart rate is already low** or we're keeping a close eye on their well-being.

So it's best in **early or mid-labour** – not just before pushing.

WATER: THE UNDERRATED HERO

Water is honestly one of the most underrated forms of pain relief in labour. You don't even need to give birth in it to feel the benefits – just *being* in warm water can be a game-changer. It calms your nervous system, helps relax your muscles, lowers adrenaline and gives your body space to soften into the process.

One woman wanted me to hold the shower head over her belly every time she had a contraction. We did that for the *entire* labour. She gave birth using **just that**. No meds. Just warm water on her stomach, every time she felt a wave coming. I've had others sit in a birth pool while their partner pours water over their back or belly with a bowl, like a little spa moment. It sounds simple, but **don't sleep on it**. It keeps you grounded, it keeps you breathing, it keeps you *calm*. You can still use **gas and air while in the water**. You don't have to pick one. Stack your tools.

Now, if you're the kind of babe who already knows, 'Yeah, no – I'm going *straight* for that epidural,' babe, don't worry about the water. Keep your clothes on, and tell them to get the anaesthetist ready. No shame. But if you're hoping to stay off meds or delay them? **Water is your best friend.**

THE BIG PUSH (LITERALLY)

EPIDURAL: THE PAIN RELIEF THAT SPLITS THE ROOM

An epidural is a local anaesthetic injected into the space around your spinal cord. It blocks the pain from your waist down. You'll usually need to:

- Sit still while it's placed.
- Get a catheter because you won't feel when you need a wee.
- Stay on the bed once it's in (though 'walking epidurals' exist in theory, they're rare and don't take all the pain away).

Here's what it DOES do:
- Takes away most (if not all) of the pain.
- Helps you rest if you're exhausted.
- Keeps you mentally present if you were spiralling.

MYTHS AROUND EPIDURALS

- **'You'll be paralysed.'** No. Anaesthetists do this all the time. Many have worked 30–50 years and never seen a woman get paralysed.
- **'You'll get back pain for life.'** Some women say they have back pain afterwards. That's valid. But studies

I'M PREGNANT ... NOW WHAT?

> haven't found strong evidence it causes long-term back issues. And pregnancy itself can cause back pain. But you're allowed to say it didn't sit right with you.
> - **Dosage.** The pump has a lock. Press it once, press it 2,000 times, it's the same dose. I've seen women at war with the button and just had to say, 'Nothing's going in, my love.'

Bottom line: have it if you want. Don't have it if you don't. No shame.

THE BIRTH COMB AND SNITCH SOLDIERS THEORY

A comb? For pain relief? Like, what are we doing here – combing through contractions? But hear me out. There's actually solid science behind this. It's all about how your brain processes pain signals, and how you can trick it into focusing on something else. Let me explain it using my snitch soldiers analogy.

Imagine every time you feel pain, like from a contraction, 10,000 little soldiers run from your nerves to your brain, screaming: 'She's in pain! She's in pain! Do something!' Now, when you hold or squeeze a birth comb during a contraction, about 3,000 of those soldiers get sent to your *hand* instead. So only 7,000 soldiers are shouting from your belly.

THE BIG PUSH (LITERALLY)

Fewer snitches = less pain perceived.

That's why birth combs work. You squeeze it in your palm, and the pain signals get shared. Your brain gets a bit distracted. It's a simple way of messing with your pain perception, and for some people, it's an absolute game-changer.

OTHER NON-MEDICAL MVPS

Let's give flowers to the simple stuff:

- Tennis balls on the back (rolled or used for counterpressure)
- Firm back massage
- Hip squeezes
- Leaning over a birth ball
- Swaying, walking, dancing
- Aromatherapy
- Music or white noise
- Breathing techniques (slow, deep, grounding)

All of these help your nervous system settle. Birth partners: this is YOUR moment. You're not just there to eat snacks and hold the hospital bag. Get in position. Use those hands. Be the back rub king or queen you were born to be.

I'M PREGNANT ... NOW WHAT?

Pain is pain. But how you manage it is *your* call. Stack your tools. Change your mind. Use what helps you feel most like you. Don't measure your birth by pain. Measure it by strength, by choice, by how supported and informed you felt. You've got options. Pick the ones that feel right. That's power.

WHAT IF YOU WANT A DRUG-FREE BIRTH?

Let's talk about the other side of the coin, because yes, you absolutely *can* have a birth without any drugs at all. And if that's your goal, here are some real, practical tips to help you get there.

First things first – **try to stay at home as long as possible** if you're planning a hospital birth. At home, you're in your own environment, feeling safe and relaxed, which can make a huge difference. The truth is, the longer you're in the comfort of your own space, the less likely you are to opt for pain relief you didn't originally want. Hospitals can be busy and clinical, and just being there can make you feel like you 'should' take something even if you were determined to go without.

Distraction is your friend! Let me tell you a story: one of my friends came over to my house when she was at term. She was just a little too happy that I'm a midwife. She came closer to her due date, and we knew she'd be more comfortable at home for as long as possible. So what did we do? We turned to her favourite thing: K-dramas. We made sure she

THE BIG PUSH (LITERALLY)

had her favourite K-dramas lined up, and we even saved the last season for her to watch during labour because we knew how well it would distract her. It worked. Watching those shows, laughing, crying and getting into the story helped her manage the early labour surges beautifully without feeling like she had to rush to hospital.

Move, breathe, trust your instincts. Staying upright, swaying your hips and using deep, calming breaths all help your body to open up and keep things moving.

Create your own calm environment. Whether it's soft music, low lighting or even just your favourite cosy blanket – feeling safe and secure is key.

Have people around you who trust your plan. I've seen so many women end up taking pain relief they didn't really want, simply because they had someone in the room – a partner, a family member – who wasn't fully on board with their plan. If the people around you don't believe in what you're trying to do, it can be so easy to doubt yourself in the heat of the moment. So please, make sure whoever's with you understands your goal for a drug-free birth. Make sure they're there to **support** and **encourage** you, not to push you towards interventions unless *you* ask for them. You need people who will stand beside you, not people who will plant little seeds of doubt when you're at your most vulnerable. Birth is intense. It's emotional. It's raw. You want your team to be your cheerleaders – people who believe you can do it and who will remind you of that when you need it most.

And remember: you're not 'less than' if you decide you want pain relief later. That's not failure, that's responding to what your body is telling you in the moment. But if you're aiming for a drug-free birth, trust your body. Trust your mind. And trust that it's absolutely possible.

THE STIGMA AROUND PAIN RELIEF (AND WHY WE NEED TO LET IT GO)

Let's address the big elephant in the birthing room: **the judgement.** If you *didn't* want an epidural, and you got through labour without one? **Well done.** Seriously, massive shoutout to you. That's no small feat, and your strength deserves to be recognised.

If you *did* want an epidural and got one the minute you hit 4cm? **Well done.** That was your boundary, your plan, and you advocated for yourself. That is powerful.

If you *planned* to go natural but mid-labour changed your mind and asked for all the drugs on offer? **Well done.** You made a new decision with the information and sensations you had in that moment, and that's brave.

You're all strong. You're all worthy. You all gave birth.

THE BIG PUSH (LITERALLY)

LABOUR POSITIONS: MOVE, ROCK AND ROLL

'Vagina should face the floor – let gravity help you!'

Labour isn't just about pain management – it's also about **movement**. Research consistently shows that moving and adopting upright positions can shorten labour, reduce pain and increase maternal satisfaction. Here's a breakdown of different positions, what they're good for and considerations if you're using an epidural.

UPRIGHT AND FORWARD-LEANING POSITIONS

Standing and leaning on a partner or piece of furniture
- **What it's good for:** Uses gravity to encourage baby's descent and helps the pelvis to open.
- **Research says:** Upright positions in the first stage can reduce the duration of labour by about one hour.[16]
- **Practical tip:** Rock or sway your hips – small movements, big impact.

Walking
- **What it's good for:** Promotes progress and keeps contractions regular.

- **What research says:** Even gentle movement can reduce the need for interventions like augmentation.[17]
- **Practical tip:** Don't worry about speed – a slow stroll is enough.

Hands and knees / All fours

- **What it's good for:** Relieves back pain; can help a posterior ('back-to-back') baby rotate.
- **What research says:** Positions like hands-and-knees may improve foetal rotation, although studies are mixed.[18]
- **Practical tip:** This can be especially helpful in the early and active stages of labour.

Squatting

- **What it's good for:** Maximises the pelvic diameter, particularly useful in second stage when pushing.
- **What research says:** Squatting can open the pelvic outlet by up to 30 per cent more than lying down.[19]
- **Practical tip:** Support from a partner, a squat bar or even pillows can make it more sustainable.

Lunging

- **What it's good for:** Opens the pelvis unevenly to help baby rotate.
- **What research says:** While high-quality trials are limited, clinical guidance sources (like the Mayo Clinic) list lunging as a labour position that can relieve lower back discomfort.

THE BIG PUSH (LITERALLY)

- **Practical tip:** Place one knee on a chair or bed and lunge forward – gentle and effective.

Sitting on a birth ball
- **What it's good for:** Comfort, gentle bouncing to encourage descent and good alignment for baby.
- **What research says:** Using a birth ball during labour is associated with lower pain scores, shorter labour duration and higher birth satisfaction.[20]

Practical tip: Use a ball as much as you can – have one at your house so you can use it during the early stages of labour.

SEMI-RECLINED POSITIONS

Supported sitting or semi-sitting on a bed
- **What it's good for:** Offers rest while still letting gravity play a role.
- **What research says:** Some position reviews suggest that semi-reclined or semi-sitting postures may offer a balance, giving you rest while still harnessing gravity's effect.[21]
- **Practical tip:** Lean forward slightly to really let gravity help.

Side-lying / Lateral positions lying on your side
- **What it's good for:** Rest, comfort and maintaining an open pelvis – especially if you're tired or have an epidural.

- **What research says:** Lateral positions can help avoid compressing major blood vessels and may improve oxygen flow to the baby.[22]
- **Practical tip:** A pillow between your knees can enhance comfort and alignment.

MOVEMENT ON AN EPIDURAL

Movement may be more limited, but small shifts still matter.

- **Side-lying with pillows for support:** Encourages baby's descent and rotation, while providing maximum comfort.
- **Semi-reclined or upright sitting in bed:** Even slight upright angles can make a difference in baby's progress.
- **Lateral tilt or alternating side-lying:** Switching sides every 20–30 minutes can help baby rotate if needed.
- **Use of a peanut ball:** If your hospital has one, a peanut ball between the knees or thighs in side-lying positions can help keep the pelvis open and encourage baby to move down.

WHY THESE POSITIONS MATTER

Movement in labour is not just about comfort – it's about working with your body and your baby.

THE BIG PUSH (LITERALLY)

> Upright and forward-leaning positions allow the pelvis to open, use gravity to your advantage, and help baby find the best position for birth. Lying on your back can actually narrow the pelvic space, which is why 'vagina should face the floor' is more than just a catchphrase. It's a principle that aligns with what research tells us.

BIRTH TRAUMA: WHAT IT IS AND WHY IT MATTERS

Birth trauma can be physical, like severe tearing or heavy blood loss, but often, it's emotional. It's that feeling of being out of control, unheard, disrespected or completely ignored during one of the most vulnerable moments of your life.

By definition, birth trauma refers to the distress a person feels during or after childbirth, which can lead to symptoms like flashbacks, nightmares, panic attacks or even post-traumatic stress disorder (PTSD). In the UK, approximately one in 25 women (about 30,000 women each year) develop PTSD following childbirth.[23] But let me make this clear: trauma isn't just about what happened to your body. It's about how you were treated, how you felt, and whether you felt safe and heard.

TWO BIRTH STORIES: WHY THE EMOTIONAL SIDE MATTERS

During my research, I spoke to a lot of women about their birth experiences, and two stories stood out to me. Both women gave birth, but their experiences couldn't have been more different.

Story 1: The 'Horrific' Birth That Was Still Beautiful

I spoke to one woman who, on paper, had what most people would consider a nightmare birth. She came into labour, fully dilated, ready to push, but then things took a turn. Baby started showing signs of distress. They tried a kiwi (a vacuum extraction), but it didn't work. They tried forceps, and it didn't work. She was rushed to theatre for an emergency C-section, where she ended up losing 2.5 litres of blood, which is a massive blood loss by any standard.

So to sum it up, this woman had:

- Full dilation.
- A failed kiwi.
- Failed forceps.
- Been rushed to theatre.
- An episiotomy (where they cut the perineum to help get the baby out).
- An emergency C-section.
- A loss of 2.5 litres of blood.

THE BIG PUSH (LITERALLY)

But do you know what she said to me? She said it was the most beautiful birth experience. Everyone kept her updated. They told her what was happening at every stage. They spoke to her with respect. She felt included in every decision. She felt like a person, not just a body on a table. And this woman? She said she's literally waiting for her two-year mark so she can get pregnant again because she was so happy with her birth.

Story 2: The 'Straightforward' Birth That Left Deep Scars

I spoke to a second woman, who had a vaginal birth six years ago, and to this day, she is adamant that she will never have another baby because of that birth alone. But what happened to her? Did she have a C-section? A massive tear? Severe blood loss? No. She had what most people would call a straightforward vaginal birth.

But here's what she told me:

- She felt like her consent didn't matter.
- She felt like no one told her what was happening.
- She felt ignored, disrespected and alone.
- Vaginal examinations were done without consideration, and when her baby came out, the baby wasn't crying straight away, but no one told her why.

That was six years ago, and she's still carrying that trauma with her. *Six years.* So you see? Birth trauma isn't always about what happened to your body. It's about what happened to your mind. It's about how you were treated and how you felt.

I'm not telling you this to scare you. I'm telling you this because **trauma isn't just about the physical**. It's about the **emotional** side too, and I genuinely believe there are things you can do to **reduce** the risk of birth trauma. I want to **reassure** those of you who have had vaginal births and felt traumatised. You're not alone. Trauma isn't reserved for people with complicated births or emergency C-sections. **Anyone** can be traumatised, and that doesn't make your experience any less valid.

WAYS TO REDUCE THE RISK OF BIRTH TRAUMA

While birth trauma can't always be prevented, there are things you can do to *reduce* the risk:

- **Educate Yourself.** Take **antenatal classes** (like mine, if you're up for it).
- **Learn About All the Possible Emergencies and Interventions.** Know your pain relief options, your rights and what might happen in different scenarios.
- **Choose the Right Birth Partner(s).** Pick someone who will **advocate** for you, not just someone who's

THE BIG PUSH (LITERALLY)

> good at holding a camera. Make sure they understand your birth plan and your boundaries.
> - **Speak Up for Yourself.** Don't be afraid to ask questions. If something doesn't feel right, **say it**.
> - **Make a Birth Plan (But Stay Flexible).** It's good to have a plan, but understand that things can change. That doesn't mean you failed.
> - **Debrief After the Birth.** Speak to your midwife or doctor if you felt unheard or confused about what happened. Get clarity, get support, get it off your chest.
> - **Postpartum Support.** Whether it's counselling, birth trauma support groups or just talking to someone who gets it, don't hold it all in.

SNACKS IN LABOUR: YES, YOU CAN EAT (BUT MAYBE NOT A FULL ROAST DINNER)

Some people will tell you, 'Oh, you can't eat in labour,' as if your body is supposed to run a marathon on an empty stomach. Let me make this clear: you can eat in labour. In fact, you should eat in labour, especially in the early stages. Your body is about to do one of the hardest things it will ever do, and you need energy for that.

But here's the thing – not all foods are created equal in labour. I once looked after a woman who clearly missed that memo. I was watching her eat, and I was thinking, *Hmm, she's going in a bit heavy there.* She was munching on chips, chicken and I'm pretty sure there were peas involved because one pea entered my Crocs. I literally looked at her like, *Yeah, I'm pissed.* And guess what? As predicted, she vomited everywhere. Not a cute, dainty vomit either. I'm talking everywhere. I was just standing there, bowl in hand, thinking, *This is why I said slow down.* So let's avoid that, shall we?

WHAT TO EAT IN LABOUR (WITHOUT MAKING A SCENE)

When it comes to labour snacks, you want things that will release energy slowly, keep your sugar levels stable and won't make you regret every bite when you're in the throes of transition. Here are some solid options:

- Bananas (potassium for muscle function).
- Nut butter on rice cakes.
- Oats or flapjacks (slow release carbs).
- Dried fruit (apricots, dates, raisins).
- Energy bars (just check the sugar content).
- Crackers and hummus.
- Fruit pouches or purées (easy to swallow and quick to digest).
- Smoothies (preferably homemade, with protein and slow carbs).

THE BIG PUSH (LITERALLY)

- Greek yoghurt or skyr (high in protein, low in sugar).
- Plain popcorn (light and easy to munch on).
- Trail mix (nuts, seeds, dried fruit).

WHAT TO DRINK IN LABOUR

Staying hydrated is crucial. You don't want to be that person passing out in second stage because you've sweated out every drop of fluid. Here are some good options:

- Isotonic drinks (replace electrolytes).
- Flavoured water (if plain water makes you gag).
- Diluted squash (not too sugary).
- Coconut water (natural electrolytes).
- Weak tea or herbal infusions (nothing too heavy).

FOR MY MUMMIES WITH GESTATIONAL DIABETES

I see you, my GD mummies. I know this is a bit different for you because you have to keep your sugar levels in check, even during labour. But that doesn't mean you can't snack. You just need to be smart about it. Here are some GD-friendly options:

- Nuts and seeds (healthy fats, low carb).
- Greek yoghurt or skyr (high protein, low carb).
- Cheese and whole-grain crackers.

- Veggie sticks with hummus.
- Boiled eggs (quick protein hit).
- Berries (low in sugar but packed with nutrients).
- Low-sugar protein bars (check the carb content).
- Sugar-free jelly or gelatine snacks.
- Homemade chia pudding (with unsweetened almond milk).

And for drinks:

- Water (obviously).
- Diet or sugar-free squash.
- Zero-sugar electrolyte drinks.
- Unsweetened iced tea.

WHEN YOU MIGHT NEED TO HOLD OFF ON THE SNACKS

Now, before you start packing a three-course meal for the birth centre, let's talk about when *not* to eat:

- If you're having an epidural, some hospitals will restrict your food and drink because of the small risk of needing a general anaesthetic.
- If you're going into theatre for a C-section, they'll usually ask you to stop eating beforehand.

THE BIG PUSH (LITERALLY)

- If you're nauseous or already vomiting, maybe stick to liquids or light snacks.

Push Past the 'I'm Not Hungry'

Now, I know some of you are going to be like, 'But I'm not hungry.' If that's the only reason you're not eating, push past it. You're about to run a marathon, climb a mountain and lift a car all at the same time. You're going to need energy for that. You need the fuel to keep your muscles moving, your brain sharp and your body pushing. Even if you're not hungry, nibble on something. Get those carbs in. You'll thank yourself later when you're in the thick of it and still have a bit of energy left in the tank.

WHEN TO GO TO THE HOSPITAL (AND WHEN TO STAY PUT)

This isn't a one-size-fits-all situation. I could give you all the tips, tricks and hacks, but on the day, you are the best judge of what your body needs. That said, there are a few guidelines you should keep in mind, and it starts with knowing what your specific hospital wants you to do.

Know Your Hospital's Protocol: Every hospital is different. Some want you to call the minute you feel your first contraction, while others are happy for you to hang out at home until things really heat up. So, step one is to find out what your hospital's policy is. Do they want you to call as soon as your waters break?

Do they want you to come in if you're having regular contractions, or just call first? Do they have specific advice for second- or third-time mums? Call them, check their website or ask your midwife. Knowledge is power.

WHEN YOUR WATERS BREAK

All right, let's get into one of the big ones: when your waters break. Here's what to do if this happens:

- **Note the Time.** It doesn't have to be precise, like '3:32 p.m.,' but a rough idea, like 'around 5:30', is helpful.
- **Check the Colour.** Is it clear, pale or tinged with a bit of blood (normal)? Or is it green, yellow or brown (not normal)?
- **Smell It.** It has a very distinctive smell – can't necessarily describe it, but if it smells foul or strong, that's a red flag.
- **Call the Hospital.** Some hospitals will ask you to come in straight away, while others might tell you to stay put and wait for contractions to kick in.

When to Go In Straight Away:
- If your waters are green, yellow or brown (possible meconium, meaning baby might be in distress).

THE BIG PUSH (LITERALLY)

- If you're pre-term (before 37 weeks).
- If you're having reduced foetal movements.
- If you have a fever or feel generally unwell.

What to Do If You Start Contractions: If you're trying to avoid an epidural or a cascade of interventions, you might want to stay home a bit longer. I always say, the hospital is a service, and the longer you're there, the more interventions you are likely to be offered. Your body is more likely to relax at home, which means better oxytocin and more efficient contractions.

My Personal Rule: Go to the hospital if you're contracting consistently – not this 'twice now and then nothing for an hour' business. If you're having two to three contractions every 10 minutes, each lasting about 40 seconds, and this pattern has been consistent for four to five hours, you are very likely in labour.

But here's the important part: this isn't about waiting a set number of hours before you're 'allowed' to call your midwife or go to hospital. It's about recognising a steady, reliable pattern instead of reacting to a few early contractions. Many providers use a similar rule of thumb, looking for contractions every three to five minutes, lasting 30 to 60 seconds. Both are simply ways of saying the same thing: once your contractions are regular, strong and not going away, labour has probably begun.

If you can keep this up at home, by the time you get to the hospital, you're probably in active labour and not going to be sent home. I've heard all the stories of women being sent home at 2cm, only to race back an hour later fully dilated. That's not because the midwife was wrong about your cervix. It's because your body can close up in a clinical setting, only to kick back in when you're back in your safe space.

If you're having a home birth, your community midwife should have already told you when to call them, what to expect and what their specific rules are. If you are ever unsure, or if you feel worried at any point, always call your midwife or maternity unit. Trust your instincts. This guideline is here to help you recognise the rhythm of labour, not to stop you from getting help when you need it.

WHEN TO GO IN STRAIGHT AWAY (EMERGENCIES)

Of course, there are **exceptions** to the 'wait it out at home' rule. If any of these things happen, you need to **go in immediately**:

- **Heavy Vaginal Bleeding.** Not just a bit of bloody show, but **heavy** bleeding like a period.
- **Green, Yellow or Brown Waters.** As I said earlier, this could mean **meconium.**
- **Reduced or No Foetal Movements.** If baby has gone quiet, that's a **big** red flag.
- **Constant, Severe Abdominal Pain.** Not like contractions that come and go, but constant pain that doesn't ease up.

THE BIG PUSH (LITERALLY)

- **Severe Headache or Blurry Vision.** Could be a sign of **pre-eclampsia**.
- **Sudden, Severe Swelling of Your Hands, Feet or Face.** Another possible sign of pre-eclampsia.
- **Fluid That Smells Foul or Feels Hot.** Could be an infection.
- **High Fever or Chills.** Not normal in labour.
- **Sudden, Sharp Chest Pain or Shortness of Breath.** Get checked out, please.

> ### AMBULANCE DRAMA
>
> I was on my break, eating my prawn cocktail crisps, relaxed, minding my own business, as I do. Then, out of nowhere, the double doors bang open, like a scene out of *Grey's Anatomy*. I look up, and I see a trolley coming through with an ambulance crew, all serious, rushing in like we're about to do a heart transplant. I'm like, *What in the world is this? What's going on?*
>
> One of the paramedics says, 'She's having contractions.' So, I took her into a room, reassured her that she was in safe hands, and asked for her consent to do a vaginal examination. She agreed, so I checked her, and she was 1cm. One. I told her, 'You're 1cm,' and that we'd advise her to go back home and continue her early labour there, where she'd probably be more comfortable and relaxed. And she just let out this big sigh, like, 'Oh, okay.'

> Just chilled. The tension left her body so fast, you'd think I just told her she won the lottery. She came in by ambulance and then left on the bus. So, please, have your travel sorted. Get a taxi, call a friend, walk if you can, but maybe skip the 999 call if it's just contractions.

WHEN TO GO TO THE HOSPITAL

Second-Time (or More) Mamas

All right, if this isn't your first rodeo, the 'wait it out' advice might not work for you. Second-time mamas, third-time mamas, and those who've had precipitate labours (those fast and furious ones that make you feel like you're starring in a Netflix special) have different things to consider.

You've done this before. You've pushed, you've breathed, you've birthed. You know that your body has muscle memory, and sometimes that means things can move a lot faster the second (or third or fourth) time around, especially if your previous births were delivered vaginally.

Signs You Should Head In a Bit Sooner:
- Your contractions are coming hard and fast right from the start.
- You're feeling a lot of pressure down below.
- You're getting that 'I need to push' feeling earlier than expected.

THE BIG PUSH (LITERALLY)

- You're already 3-4cm dilated at your last check (some of you walk around like this for weeks).

Basically, if your first baby took 12 hours, don't assume your second will take the same amount of time. Be prepared to move faster.

For My Precipitate Labour Mamas

If you've had a precipitate (rapid) labour before, you already know what this is like. These are the mamas who go from zero to baby in three hours or less. If this is you, you don't have time to be faffing around. Consider:

- Going in as soon as you feel regular contractions, even if they're not that strong yet.
- Making sure your bag is packed and ready to grab and go.
- Having a backup plan for childcare if you've got other little ones at home.
- Considering a home birth if you're low risk and your team is on board, so you don't end up giving birth on the A406.

Other Reasons to Go In Sooner If This Isn't Your First Baby:
- **Fast Progression Last Time.** If you hit active labour quickly with your first, you might do the same again.

- **High Pain Threshold.** If you were one of those 'I didn't feel much until I was 8cm' mamas the first time, don't push your luck.
- **Big Babies.** If you've had a big baby before and you're feeling a lot of pressure early on, maybe don't wait until you're crowning.
- **Gut Feeling.** You know your body. If it's telling you to go in, go in.

VBAC Mamas

If you're planning a VBAC, first of all, big respect. I know it's not always an easy choice, and you've probably had to advocate for this birth plan, so I'm rooting for you. But let's talk about when to head in, because it's a bit different for you.

A VBAC is an incredible option for many women, but it comes with a slightly higher risk of uterine rupture (I know, scary word, but it's rare), so your midwife or doctor is going to want to keep a closer eye on you once things kick off.

When to Go In If You're Having a VBAC:
- **Early, Consistent Contractions.** As soon as you feel regular contractions, even if they're mild, it's a good idea to go in.
- **Sharp, Sudden Pain.** If you feel a sharp, tearing pain or something doesn't feel right, go in immediately.

THE BIG PUSH (LITERALLY)

- **Bleeding.** Any more than a little bloody show or spotting should be checked out.
- **Change in Baby's Movements.** If you notice a sudden drop in baby's movements, don't wait.
- **Severe Pressure or Intense Pain at Your Scar.** This one's big. If you feel a burning or tearing sensation around your previous C-section scar, get to the hospital straight away.
- **Gut Feeling.** I know I keep saying this, but trust your instincts. You know your body, and if something feels off, go in.

When you arrive, they'll likely want to:

- **Monitor Baby's Heart Rate.** Just to make sure they're handling the contractions well.
- **Check Your Scar Area.** To make sure there's no unusual tenderness or pressure.
- **Keep a Closer Eye on You.** Don't be surprised if they want to keep you in once you arrive. That's just them being extra cautious.

Tips for a Smoother VBAC Hospital Arrival:

- **Bring Your Birth Plan.** Make sure everyone knows this is a VBAC.
- **Advocate for Movement.** Just because you're being monitored doesn't mean you have to be flat on your back.

I'M PREGNANT ... NOW WHAT?

BIRTH PARTNERS

I've been excited to talk about birth partners because I genuinely feel like I've seen it all. I've seen grandmothers that swear they did it all alone in their day, squatting in a field without so much as a paracetamol. I've seen the birth partners that make you want to hug them and the ones that make you want to kick them out. I've had birth partners:

- **Nap on the Bed.** While the mum is on the floor, contracting, fighting for her life.
- **Ask for an ETA.** One birth partner actually asked me, 'How long is this going to take? I've got somewhere to be.' What?
- **Leave at 8cm.** I once had a birth partner go home when the woman was 8cm because they were exhausted. The cheek.

But on the flip side, I've also seen some incredible birth partners. The ones that make you think, *Hmm, maybe my standards need to go up.* I've seen birth partners who:

- **Hold Their Partners Up.** Literally hold them up through every contraction.
- **Breathe with Them.** Matching every breath, counting every push, never breaking eye contact.

THE BIG PUSH (LITERALLY)

- **Advocate Like a Lawyer.** Asking all the right questions, making sure their partner's voice is heard.
- **Keep the Vibes Right.** Playing the right music, keeping the energy in the room calm and positive.
- **Keep Mum Laughing.** Cracking jokes between contractions, keeping the mood light.

Honestly, I feel so sorry for my future husband, because I've seen greatness in that delivery room, and now my standards are high.

PICK SOMEONE WHO LOVES YOU, BUT KNOWS HOW TO HOLD IT TOGETHER

Now, of course, you want someone who loves you in that room. That's a given. But there's a certain type of love you need in the delivery room. You need someone who can hold it down when things get real. Someone who can keep their emotions in check when yours are all over the place.

I've seen birth partners break down in tears, and I get it. It's emotional. It's intense. But you don't need someone crying harder than you when you're the one pushing a whole human out. This is the kind of person you want:

- **The Rock.** Someone who can be your calm in the storm, not someone who falls apart when the contractions start rolling in.

- **The Encourager.** Someone who can lift you up when you're ready to give up, but also knows when to just shut up and hold your hand.
- **The Steady Hand.** Someone who won't panic if things get intense, who can keep you grounded when you're spiralling.

It's not about picking the person who loves you the most, but the person who can show up for you in a way that's calm, strong and reassuring. Because in that moment, you don't need drama – you need support.

YOUR PARTNER ISN'T ALWAYS THE BEST CHOICE

Just because someone is the father of your child doesn't necessarily mean they're the best birth partner for you. This goes for all kinds of relationships – whether it's your husband, boyfriend, wife, partner or anyone else you share your life with. Some people know, deep down, that their partner isn't built for the chaos of the delivery room. And that's okay. That doesn't make them any less of a great partner or parent.

I've seen it all. I've seen partners who step up and become birth legends. I've seen the ones whose eyes go wide when they realise just how powerful their partner is. I've seen the ones who come out the other side with a deeper bond, new-found respect and a whole new level of admiration for the

THE BIG PUSH (LITERALLY)

person they love. But I've also seen the ones who just can't handle it. The ones who panic, faint or just shut down under pressure. If that's your partner, you need to ask yourself, 'Is this going to help me or stress me out?'

You want someone in the room who's going to calm you, centre you and encourage you. Not someone who's going to make you worry about their well-being when you should be focusing on your own. I've even seen a woman have her neighbour as her birth partner, and it was a beautiful birth. She said her neighbour was just calm, reassuring and steady – exactly what she needed.

And this whole idea of, 'Oh, it'll make my husband (or partner) understand what we go through and value us more,' is a bit of a trap. Your partner should be valuing you regardless. They shouldn't need to watch you push a whole human out to understand your strength.

HOW TO SPOT A GREAT BIRTH PARTNER (HINT: NOT EVERYONE IS A MARY OR A WUNMI)

I went to Malta for my friend's hen do, and we ended up on this boat trip. Now, let me tell you, the motion sickness was beating me up. I was going through it, vomiting, feeling like the waves were winning the fight. There was the bride's sister, Mary and her cousin, Wunmi – those two were amazing.

Mary quietly handed me a vomit bag, checked in on me, made sure I had space to breathe and compose myself, but also stayed close enough that I knew she had my back. Wunmi was right there too, keeping the vibes in check, making sure I had everything I needed, and never hovering or making me feel smothered. They were just solid. In that moment, I thought, 'Wow, you two would make amazing birth partners.'

Then, there was Nini. Bless her heart. She was trying to be supportive, giving me words of encouragement, but the minute she saw me vomit, her empathy kicked in, and she started gagging too. You know those ones who are just a bit too sensitive to handle the messy side of things? That's Nini. Then there was Titi. Listen, Titi was already fighting for her life downstairs. She was the first to start vomiting, way before I even felt a twinge. She was on the ropes before the boat even hit a wave.

And it made me realise something: in the delivery room, you want a Mary or a Wunmi - someone who can hold it down, keep calm and support you without falling apart. A Nini might have the best intentions, but if she's going to pass out at the sight of an epidural or start gagging when you're trying to push, she might not be the best choice. And a Titi? You don't want someone who's struggling with their own trauma or fighting for their life in the corner when you're trying to bring life into the world.

So when you're picking a birth partner, look for the Marys and Wunmis in your life - the ones who can hold it together, keep you calm and support you without making it about themselves. Because trust me, when things get real, you don't want to be the one comforting your birth partner.

> ### THE GRANDMA DILEMMA
>
> If I could BAN future grandmas from the birth room, I would. Okay, so obviously not *all* grandmas – I've seen phenomenal ones. But I've also seen grandmas who can't cope with their daughter being in pain. They'll say things like, 'Oh my gosh, you're not going to have an epidural?' or 'In my day, we just had to get on with it.' And you don't want to feel like you've failed in your birth because someone in the room can't handle their own emotions.
>
> At the end of the day, your birth partner should be someone who brings you peace, not pressure. Someone who can centre you, calm you and hold it down when things get real. Whether it's your partner, your mum, your best friend or even your neighbour, choose someone who can handle the chaos without falling apart, someone who will advocate for you when you need it, and someone who knows how to support without smothering. In that delivery room, you deserve to feel safe, loved and fully supported.

I'M PREGNANT ... NOW WHAT?

BIRTH ROOM ENERGY: IT DOESN'T HAVE TO BE A WAR ZONE

Movies have lied to us, honestly. They make it seem like every woman in labour has to scream, swear and shout at their partner like it's a battlefield. The whole, 'You did this to me!' vibe. But it doesn't have to be like that. This is the person you love, the one you've decided to bring life into this world with. Your baby is a symbol of your love, so that energy should still be there, even in the chaos.

Yes, you're in pain. Yes, you might get irritated. Yes, you might snap at times, and that's okay. But it doesn't have to be pure aggression. I've seen women come in with their partners and shut them down so hard that you'd think they were enemies. But I've also seen the ones who breathe together, lock eyes and support each other like they're the only two people in the world.

Here's how you can keep that **love** at the centre of it all:

- **Involve Them Early.** Don't wait until you're 10cm to start telling them what you need. Include them in the birth plan, let them know your preferences and talk about pain relief options together.
- **Empower Them to Advocate.** You shouldn't have to repeat yourself when you're in the middle of a contraction. If you've already told your partner you

don't want a certain intervention, they should be able to step up and say it on your behalf.
- **Talk About Expectations.** Let them know that, yes, you might snap, but it's not personal. And also, it doesn't have to be a scream fest. They can be your calm when you're feeling overwhelmed.
- **Give Them a Role.** Whether it's massaging your back, counting your breaths or just being the one to hold you, give them a job so they feel useful and not like a spare part.
- **Remember the Love.** This baby is a product of your love. It doesn't have to feel like a battle to bring them into the world.
- **Plan for the Little Things.** What if someone asks you a question while you're contracting? They should have the answer. That way, you're not being bombarded when you're just trying to breathe.

At the end of the day, the birth room can be a place of connection, not conflict. It's where you'll meet your baby for the first time, where you'll see your partner step up in ways you didn't even know they could.

So, if you can, keep that love at the centre of it all. It will make the whole experience sweeter.

I'M PREGNANT ... NOW WHAT?

DEAR BIRTH PARTNER – THIS BIT IS FOR YOU

All right, so ideally, I'd want you to read the whole book, but I get it – if you can't, at least take a moment to read this. You'll hear a lot of people say: *It's not about you.* The day isn't about you. The baby isn't about you. It's all about the mum. And yes, it is about the mum, but hear me out – it's also about you. You're a key part of this day.

I've seen birth partners make or break a birth. I've seen women that won't listen to a word I say until their birth partner says it. I've seen labour speed up just because a partner got the vibes right. I've seen a calm, supportive birth partner change the entire energy of a room. So don't ever let anyone tell you that you're not important. You are.

I think it's just the shitty birth partners that have ruined it for the rest of you. You know the ones who come in checking football scores, fall asleep on the bed or moan about the hospital WiFi? Yeah. Them. But if you've got this chapter in your hand, I'm assuming you're not one of them. I'm assuming you're one of the good ones.

THE BIG PUSH (LITERALLY)

PRACTICAL ADVICE FOR THE BIG DAY

- **Know Your Limits.** If you're the type to faint at the sight of a needle or blood, it's okay to stand by her head and just hold her hand. You don't have to watch the baby crown if you're not ready for that. And please – if you need a breather, step out. It's better to reset than to collapse in the room.
- **Do Your Research.** Learn a few massage techniques. Figure out how to counterpressure her back if she's having back labour. Know what positions might help her feel more comfortable. If she loves a certain show or playlist, have that queued up for those early labour hours.
- **Read the Room.** Sometimes, you'll try something and she'll love it. Other times, you'll try something and she'll hate it. That's okay. Trial and error is part of this. If she's not saying anything, it might just be because she's too tired to speak – so if she's not shoving you away, keep going.
- **Stay Engaged.** Don't get comfortable with the pain. I've noticed that some birth partners start out strong – rubbing backs, whispering encouragement, holding hands – but as the hours go by, they start to fade. They get used to the sounds of pain and think it's

normal now, so they back off. Don't. That's when you need to dig deep and double down. Be that PT that keeps someone on the treadmill for those last 10 minutes, not the one who lets them coast.

- **Focus on What You Can Do, Not What You Can't.** There's going to come a moment in that room when it all feels too much. You're going to see her in pain, you're going to feel helpless, and you're going to want to fix it, but you can't. In those moments, it's easy to shut down, pull away or even snap out of frustration. But don't. Focus on what you can do: hand her an ice drink, fan her, whisper words of affirmation, squeeze her hand, remind her of her strength. It might seem small, but those little things matter.

WORDS OF ENCOURAGEMENT

Listen, I know this isn't easy. It's a lot of pressure, but trust me, you're important. I've seen women breathe easier just because their partner whispered the right words at the right time. I've seen pain become manageable because a partner was consistent with that back rub or kept reassuring them through the contractions. Don't ever let anyone make you feel like you're not a big part of this process. You are.

THE BIG PUSH (LITERALLY)

> **You Are the Difference**
>
> You are the one who can steady a shaky room. You are the one who can bring calm to the chaos. You are the one who can help make this birth a beautiful experience. So show up, stay present and keep going – even when you think they've got used to the pain, keep going. You might be the reason they push through.

REASONS YOU MIGHT STAY IN HOSPITAL LONGER

We'd love for you to be able to head home as soon as you and baby are fine, baby's feeding well, and you're both settled. I'm a big believer in the power of being in your own space, with your things and your people. And listen, it really can be that quick for some people.

I remember one mum who came in super early in the morning – her second baby, so she knew what to expect. She dropped her first child off at breakfast club, came into the hospital around 7 a.m., and was back in time to pick them up at after-school club. She was buzzing, like, 'Oh my gosh, I can't believe it! I left pregnant, came back with a baby.' But it's not like that for everyone.

Some people stay in the hospital so long that I start thinking they could recite my shift pattern better than I could. Some babies take their time settling into this world, some recoveries take a bit longer, and sometimes, we just want to monitor a few things before sending you home. It's not always because something is wrong – sometimes it's just about precaution, support or recovery. So, let's talk about the reasons you might end up staying a bit longer – for mummy and baby.

Mummy Reasons

- **Heavy Bleeding (Postpartum Haemorrhage).** If you had a heavy bleed during or after birth, we might need to monitor you a bit longer to make sure you're stable and your iron levels are okay.
- **Surgery Recovery (C-Section).** If you had a C-section, you'll need time to recover, get your pain under control, and make sure the incision is healing well.
- **High Blood Pressure (Pre-eclampsia or Eclampsia).** If you had high blood pressure during pregnancy, we might need to keep an eye on you to make sure it settles after birth.
- **Infections (Sepsis or Wound Infections).** If you develop an infection or if you had a tear that got infected, we'll need to keep you in for antibiotics and monitoring.
- **Post-Operative Monitoring.** If you had any complications during birth, like a forceps delivery or vacuum extraction, you might need to stay a bit longer for observation.
- **Mental Health Support.** If you're feeling overwhelmed, anxious or struggling with your mental health, we might keep you in for some extra support.

THE BIG PUSH (LITERALLY)

- **Excessive Pain.** If your pain isn't being well controlled, it's better to stay where we can adjust your meds and keep an eye on you.
- **Retained Placenta or Clots.** If the placenta didn't come away cleanly or if you have clots that won't clear, you might need to stay for treatment.
- **Mobility Issues.** If you're struggling to move after birth, we might keep you in to monitor your recovery and help you mobilise safely.

Baby Reasons

- **Feeding Challenges.** If baby is struggling to latch, feed or gain weight, we might need to keep you both in for a bit longer to establish breastfeeding or support with bottle feeding.
- **Jaundice.** If baby is looking a bit yellow, they might need phototherapy to break down the excess bilirubin in their system.
- **Low Blood Sugar (Hypoglycaemia).** If baby has low blood sugar, they might need a bit more monitoring and possibly top-up feeds to stabilise their levels.
- **Breathing Difficulties.** If baby is having a bit of trouble breathing or their oxygen levels are low, they might need some extra support.
- **Infection (Sepsis).** If baby shows any signs of infection, they might need antibiotics and monitoring for a few days.

- **Temperature Regulation.** If baby is struggling to maintain their temperature, we might keep them in to make sure they're staying warm enough.
- **Blood Incompatibility (Rhesus Factor Issues).** If there's a blood type mismatch, baby might need a bit more monitoring for jaundice or anaemia.
- **Prematurity.** If baby arrived a bit early, they might need a bit more support to feed, regulate their temperature and grow.
- **Observations for Meconium Aspiration.** If baby passed meconium (poo) in the womb, we might need to monitor them for breathing difficulties.
- **Birth Trauma or Injuries.** If baby had a difficult birth, like a forceps delivery or shoulder dystocia, they might need a bit more observation.
- **Low Birth Weight.** If baby is smaller than expected, we might need to keep them in for a few days to monitor their weight gain and ensure they're feeding well. This might also mean a day-three weight check.

So, while some people are in and out in a matter of hours, others need a bit more time to settle in, recover and adjust. It's not a race, and it's not a competition. Whether you're one of the ones who dashes in and out, or the one who knows all my shift patterns by the end, the goal is to make sure you and baby are safe, healthy and ready for the next chapter at home.

PART 5

POSTPARTUM

YOUR BODY, YOUR BABY, YOUR NEW NORMAL

This book is literally called *I'm Pregnant ... Now What?* and the plan was to focus on pregnancy. But let me be honest with you: it would be absolutely criminal if I didn't speak about the postnatal stage. Why? Because this is the part where so many mums get forgotten. It's the bit where people stop checking in, stop asking how *you* are, and shift their attention entirely to the baby. And the last thing I ever want to do is make you feel unseen.

Now, if you're reading this as a second-time mum, this might be the section where things click differently. You might find yourself thinking, 'Ahh, if only I'd known this the first time around ...' That's why I couldn't leave this part out. I can't in good conscience finish a book on pregnancy and just pat you on the back like, 'Well done, good luck!' That would be mad.

As a midwife, I usually only get to care for women for the first 28 days after birth. But even in those few short weeks, so much happens - emotionally, physically, mentally - and not enough people are talking about it in a way that feels honest. I want to talk to you about the reality of that first wee, the kind that makes you hold your breath and question everything. I want to talk about what baby blues really feel like, what postnatal depression can look like and how sometimes you don't realise you need help until you're already drowning. I want to talk about the check-ups that get missed, the bits of you that feel broken or unrecognisable, the way birth trauma can sneak up on you, and even the everyday stuff, like how to clean your baby's cord stump.

POSTPARTUM EMOTIONAL RECOVERY

Postpartum is the single biggest hormonal crash in human biology. Bigger than puberty. Bigger than menopause. And yet, no one really prepares you for it. One minute you're riding the high of birth, the next you're crying over toast, spiralling because you can't remember the last time you showered, and wondering if you're doing anything right.

We're going to start with Mummy. I always say I'm a midwife, and that literally means 'with woman' - that's where my focus is. That's where my heart is. I love babies, I really do. The little feet, the smell, all of it - but I love

POSTPARTUM

mummies more. For me, it's always been about her. About *you*. So before we get into the baby stuff, before we start talking about feeding, crying, nappies, all of that, I want to talk about *you*. The emotional shifts, the physical healing, the mental toll. If Mummy's not doing well, then baby's not doing well. Simple as that.

Let me start by saying this: you're doing better than you think. I know it might not feel like it, especially if you're running on crumbs of sleep and questioning everything, but the fact that you're even here, reading this, trying to understand yourself better, means you care. It means you're showing up. Whether you're already deep in the fourth trimester or just reading ahead to prepare yourself for what's coming, that alone matters more than anything.

So many women are still struggling silently because we've normalised suffering. We tell mums it's meant to be hard. We romanticise exhaustion and call it strength. We hand out 'supermum' badges while quietly ignoring the red flags. The truth is, you can love your baby with everything in you and still feel like you're falling apart. But when the world only celebrates the image of a glowing mum with a sleeping baby, it becomes harder and harder to say, 'I'm not okay.'

And culturally, it gets even trickier. In so many communities, especially Black and Brown ones, there's this unspoken pressure to just 'get on with it'. You're expected to be strong, to be grateful, to hold everything together. There's stigma around mental health, around medication, around even saying you're feeling low. What stings is that often those same communities won't even praise you when you're doing well, but the second something goes wrong, the judgement comes in heavy. The whispers start. The shame creeps in. Black women especially are expected to perform strength, to be unshakeable, unbreakable, unmoved. So when you don't match that impossible image, it doesn't just feel like you're struggling – it feels like you've failed.

But you haven't. You're not the failure. The way society is set up? *That's* the failure. People spend your whole pregnancy telling you, 'Just wait till the baby comes, it gets worse.' Like they're preparing you for battle instead of showing you how to heal. Then when it *does* get hard, no one's there. The same society that builds the pressure gives you nothing to hold onto when the cracks start showing.

Joy and chaos can and will coexist. I say this all the time because I truly believe the world would be a better place if more people understood that *two things can be true at the same time.* It's no different when it comes to the postnatal experience. You can have a baby who sleeps well, barely cries, feeds like a dream, and *still* feel low. Or you can be in the thick of absolute madness – cluster feeding, sore nipples, leaking through your top, no sleep in sight, and *still* feel joy bubbling up in the middle of it. Postnatal doesn't have to be one thing. It doesn't have to be awful for it to be valid, and it doesn't have to be perfect to be beautiful. I never want to be the person who paints postnatal life as one long horror story, because that's just as unhelpful as pretending everything is perfect. I've seen women go through postnatal

POSTPARTUM

periods that were full of peace, laughter and bonding, and they are just as real and just as worthy of being heard. But I've also seen women fall apart silently behind the scenes while everyone told them how 'lucky' they were. You can have a week that feels incredible and then the next week could floor you. And that doesn't make you inconsistent. Two things can be true. Always.

So how do you know when it's more than just 'new mum tired'? You start by checking in with yourself. If the low mood lasts longer than two weeks, if you're crying every day, struggling to bond with your baby, feeling numb, anxious or having thoughts that scare you, it's time to talk to someone. If you're not eating, not sleeping even when the baby is, or if your thoughts feel dark, intrusive or out of character, please, don't brush it off. You don't have to wait for it to get unbearable. You don't have to earn help by breaking down.

So let's break it down, plain and clear:

Baby blues: This usually kicks in around days three to five after birth. You might feel weepy, overwhelmed, irritable or just 'not yourself'. It's hormonal, it's common, and it typically fades within two weeks. You don't need treatment, just rest, support and people around you who get it.

Postnatal depression: This goes deeper and lasts longer. You might feel persistently low, detached, guilty, anxious or like you're failing, even when you're trying your best. You might cry daily, struggle to sleep or eat, or feel like you're not bonding with your baby. This isn't your fault – but it *is* your sign to speak to someone. Your GP, health visitor, midwife, anyone. Treatment works. Support helps.

Postnatal psychosis: This is rare, but serious. It can come on suddenly, often within the first two weeks, and may include hallucinations, delusions, confusion, paranoia or extreme mood swings. It's a medical emergency and needs immediate care. This isn't 'going mad', and it's not something you can just push through. If you or someone around you notices anything that feels 'off' or unsafe, get urgent help fast.

Each of these needs something different – but none of them make you a bad mum.

PHYSICAL RECOVERY

So we've talked about labour, we've talked about birth, but what happens *immediately* after? The baby's out, everyone's clapping, and now what? Because this part, right here, is where a lot of people feel caught off guard. You spend so much time preparing for the birth that no one really tells you what's coming in the hours, days and weeks afterwards. And let me tell you, your body is *doing a lot.*

Let's start with **lochia**, because no one talks about it enough. Lochia is the bleeding you get after you give birth. It's your body's way of clearing out everything it built up during pregnancy – blood, tissue, mucus. It's not just 'like a period', it's its own thing. Depending on your body, your

POSTPARTUM

birth and your recovery, it can last anywhere from a few weeks to even six weeks or more. At first, it can be heavy - like, *really* heavy. We're talking maternity pads, not your everyday liners. Some days it can gush a bit when you stand up or feed your baby, which can feel alarming, but it's normal. And just when you think it's stopped? Surprise. It might start again. This doesn't always mean something's wrong; your body doesn't bleed in neat little chapters. One of my friends spotted on and off for *months*. My mum said she didn't bleed at all after six weeks and didn't see a drop of blood again for another 18 months. Everyone's different, and there's no one right way to bleed.

Now let's talk **stitches**, because whew, the misconceptions! People hear 'stitches' and they imagine metal staples or something out of a horror film. But no. Most women who tear or have an episiotomy during birth are given a continuous *dissolvable* stitch. It's not a bunch of separate pieces of thread, it's one long stitch gently woven in and out, like someone sewing through soft fabric. It holds everything together neatly and dissolves on its own over time. No one's going in later to take anything out. Unless there are complications or signs of infection, you don't need to mess with it. What it really needs is *water;* clean, running water to rinse gently, and for the area to be kept dry afterwards. No scrubbing, no special soaps, no fancy products. Just water and air.

Rest is another one. We hear it all the time: 'rest for six weeks, you've just had a baby!' The justification people love to give is that you have a dinner plate-sized wound where the placenta came away from the uterus. I've heard this so many times, and while I get the sentiment behind it, it's a little off. If you had a literal dinner plate-sized wound in your uterus, you would not be here to read this. But here's the thing: *you shouldn't have to exaggerate the damage to justify needing rest.* You need rest because you just gave birth. That alone is enough. You've stretched, pushed, possibly torn, possibly been cut. You've delivered a whole human. That's major. You don't need a dramatic analogy to make your healing valid.

Let's talk **soreness and pain relief**. Depending on your birth, your body might feel like it's been hit by a truck. Muscles ache, your back might hurt, your pelvic floor might feel like it's gone on strike. If you had stitches, you might be sore when sitting or walking. For that, pain relief is your best friend. Hospitals will usually give you what you need: paracetamol, ibuprofen and, in some cases, something stronger. Now, here's one that surprises people every time: if you had stitches, you might be given a *suppository* (pain relief that goes up your bum). Yes, you read that right, and let me tell you: it is a *godsend*. It works quickly, it's effective and if they offer it to you, take it. Don't overthink it, just take it and thank yourself later.

Did you know that contractions don't actually stop after you birth the placenta? Yep, they can carry on for *days*. Welcome to the part nobody talks about: **afterpains**. Just when you think you've made it through the hardest part, your uterus says, 'Hold on, I'm not done yet,' and keeps contracting. And

POSTPARTUM

while it might sound a bit unfair, especially after everything you've just been through, it's actually your body doing exactly what it needs to do.

Afterpains are your uterus working hard to shrink back down to its pre-pregnancy size. Think of it like a big balloon deflating – it doesn't just snap back. It has to tighten and contract, again and again, to reduce in size and stop bleeding. Here's the kicker: it hurts more for some than others.

I always say life has a way of balancing things. For many **first-time mums**, labour might be longer, but they usually experience little to no afterpains – just a few twinges here and there. But for **second-time mums and beyond**, labour tends to be quicker, but the afterpains? Whew. They come in *hot*. The more babies you've had, the more intense those afterpains usually are.

Breastfeeding also turns up the volume. That's because when you breastfeed, your body releases **oxytocin**, the same hormone that causes contractions during labour. So when you're nursing your baby, your uterus is being told to tighten up again. You might notice that the cramps are strongest in those first few days, especially while feeding. They can take your breath away a bit, like a wave that rolls in right when you're trying to focus on your latch, but they *do* settle.

The good news is: they don't last forever. It's usually just the first few days that are most intense, and then it gradually calms down. It's totally normal to feel surprised by how painful they can be, especially when no one warned you.

You've done the hard bit, and now your body's doing the clean-up job.

C-SECTION RECOVERY

C-section recovery is a whole different ballgame. Sometimes it feels like the world just throws 'you had a C-section' into the mix, like it's a casual variation of birth, but let's be honest: **you've had major abdominal surgery.** If the same level of surgery had happened for any other reason, say, your appendix, you'd be on bed rest, getting served meals in bed, and probably not expected to function for weeks. But when you're a new mum? There's a baby to feed, nappies to change and a world that expects you to just crack on. So let's slow it down and talk about what recovery really needs to look like.

First off, **take it easy**. When I say 'easy', I mean *gentle*. You don't need to prove anything. You don't need to 'bounce back'. The only thing you should be lifting in those early days is your baby. That's it. Not the car seat, not the buggy, not the laundry basket – just the baby. Your body has just been through something huge, and healing well now means less chance of complications later.

The **scar** will be sore – it might feel tight or numb, and yes, in the beginning, it might ooze a little. That's completely normal. What we don't want to see are **signs of infection**: redness that's spreading, offensive smells, heat, pain that's getting worse instead of better or if it's absolutely

POSTPARTUM

leaking. If any of those are happening, it's time to call your midwife or GP.

When it comes to scar care, **keep the area clean and dry**. Gently wash it with water; no harsh soaps, no scrubbing, and pat it dry. Some women like to use a hairdryer on the cool setting to help air it out without rubbing. If you've got a bit of an overhang (which is *completely normal*), you can fold a soft muslin or pad over the top during the day to stop it getting damp or sweaty. Comfort is key.

Movement is part of recovery, but it needs to be paced. No sudden twisting. No rushing up the stairs because you 'feel fine'. I always say: just because the adrenaline is masking the pain doesn't mean the healing is done. Move slowly, listen to your body and if it hurts, stop.

One thing I always tell mums when they're preparing for baby, even if you're planning a vaginal birth, is to set your space up like you *might* need a C-section – just in case. It's not about expecting surgery or assuming the worst, but the little changes you make will benefit you either way:

- Put your nappy station on wheels.
- Keep baby's clothes and supplies at waist height.
- Use lightweight storage baskets and rolling trolleys.

These things make life easier across the board – but if you *do* end up needing a section, they become absolutely essential. You're not suddenly stuck trying to rearrange everything while healing from surgery. You've already done it.

I'M PREGNANT ... NOW WHAT?

After birth, your body goes through a significant hormonal adjustment. The drop in pregnancy hormones like oestrogen and progesterone can trigger noticeable physical symptoms, especially in the first few days. One of the most common is **night sweats**. Many women wake up drenched in sweat during the early postnatal period. It can feel intense, but it's a normal response as your body gets rid of the excess fluid and begins to regulate itself.

You might also experience **postnatal chills** – sudden episodes of shivering, even when the room is warm. These can happen soon after birth or continue in the days that follow. They're usually harmless and linked to hormonal changes and the body's recovery process. To manage these symptoms, wear breathable fabrics, keep a spare change of clothes nearby and stay hydrated. If you notice a fever, or if your chills are ongoing and severe, speak to your midwife or GP to rule out infection.

Healing looks different for every woman. Some feel okay in a few days. Some need weeks. Some need months. There's no race to 'bounce back'. In fact, I need you to unlearn that whole concept. This isn't about bouncing. This is about recovery, gentleness and listening to your body. Bleeding will stop when it stops. Stitches will dissolve when they're ready. Your body will heal if you give it the chance to. So slow down. Don't rush to be 'back to normal'. Your body did something extraordinary – and now, it deserves extraordinary care.

POSTPARTUM

THE THREE BS: BOOBS, BLADDER AND BOWELS

I know, I know. Nobody wants to talk about this part, but *this* is the real postpartum experience. It's the part that can have you googling 'how to sit without crying' at 3 a.m. or whispering 'please, please, please' to your body like it's not yours anymore.

Let's start with **boobs**, or more specifically, **engorgement**. If you're breastfeeding, or even if you're not, your milk coming in can turn your breasts into what can only be described as bricks. Hot, tight, tender bricks. Engorgement is when your breasts become overfull with milk, blood, lymph – the whole hormonal orchestra – and it can be painful. Like, *really* painful. I've seen women in tears from it. Some even say, 'I can't do this again,' because the pain blindsides them, and that heartbreak of wanting to feed your baby but feeling like your body is attacking you? It's a lot.

So what helps? First: try to **feed or express regularly**. Don't leave your breasts full for hours and hours. That fullness is what leads to engorgement. Hand express in the shower if you need to. If it's in your budget, consider seeing a **lactation consultant**. It's not always accessible, but if it's an option for you, it can be a game-changer. The difference between a cracked nipple and a confident feed can come down to one decent latch.

I'M PREGNANT ... NOW WHAT?

Now let's talk **mastitis**. This is when a blocked duct or leftover milk turns into an infection, and it's no joke. Fever, chills, flu-like symptoms and one boob that feels like it's been run over. If you feel a lump, hot area or you're in serious pain: *don't wait*. Rest, feed or express to empty the breast, apply warm compresses and speak to your GP. Antibiotics may be needed, but the best thing you can do is catch it early.

Cracked or sore nipples are really common in the early days of breastfeeding, especially while you and your baby are still figuring out the latch. The main thing is to check your positioning and latch, because most of the time that's the cause. You can also use nipple cream or expressed breast milk directly on the nipples to help them heal, and give them some air time when you can.

Next up: **peeing**. If you've had a **C-section**, you would have had a catheter, and one of the milestones we watch for is whether you've passed urine after it's been removed. We *need* to know your bladder is working again, not just because we're nosy, but because post-op swelling or pain meds can make your bladder a bit sluggish, and we don't want you walking around with a full bladder you can't feel putting pressure on your healing uterus. If you've had a vaginal birth, peeing can sting – especially if you've torn or had stitches. You might dread it. Sitting on the toilet can feel like an extreme sport. I always tell mummies: don't just let it gush out in one go. Pee a little bit, pour a little bit of warm

POSTPARTUM

water, then pee a bit more, pour again. You can use a peri bottle if you have one, or even just a clean cup of warm water. It helps dilute the urine as it passes and takes away that sharp sting. And the more hydrated you are, especially during labour, the less concentrated your urine is, which makes it sting even less. So drink up and lean forward on the toilet.

Now ... the big one. **The first poo.** No one fears poo more than someone who's just had a baby. And I don't care if it was a vaginal birth, C-section, water birth, home birth – everyone is afraid of that first one. Your core feels weak, your pelvic floor has just done a full shift and if you've had stitches, you're terrified of anything tearing or popping. I promise you: it's not as bad as you imagine.

One random – but very effective – tip? **Chew gum.** Yep. After a C-section, your bowels need to 'wake up'. Surgery, pain meds and the general shock your body's been through can slow everything down. Chewing gum helps stimulate the vagus nerve, which gets your digestive system moving again. It's simple, harmless and for some women, it makes all the difference in getting things going.

Whether it's a wee, a feed or a long-awaited poo, I just want you to know: there's nothing weird or wrong with your body right now. It's working through a lot. And you're not mad for crying because you leaked through your bra, or because the catheter made you feel like a patient when all you want to feel is like a mum.

I'M PREGNANT ... NOW WHAT?

PELVIC FLOOR RECOVERY

Let's clear this up now: **pelvic floor exercises are not just a pregnancy thing**. In fact, if you're only doing them during pregnancy and then forgetting about them once the baby arrives, you're missing the moment when they actually matter the most.

Yes, during pregnancy your pelvic floor is under pressure. But it's **after** the birth, when everything's been stretched, softened, possibly torn or even surgically adjusted, that your pelvic floor really needs support. This group of muscles helps hold up your **bladder, bowel and uterus**, and if it's weakened, it can lead to leaking, pressure or that heavy dragging feeling that so many women just accept as 'normal'. It doesn't have to be.

The good news? You don't need to carve out a whole hour of your day. You don't need gym clothes or a mat or a whole routine. Pelvic floor work is all about **consistency**, not intensity. Little and often is better than none at all. I always say: squeeze when you're brushing your teeth, feeding the baby, waiting for the kettle to boil - stack it into moments that already exist.

You can start with a **simple slow squeeze**: imagine drawing up from your back passage, as if you're trying to stop yourself passing wind. Hold for five seconds, then slowly release. Repeat that a few times. Then try some **quick pulses** - squeeze and release quickly, around 10 times. That's it.

POSTPARTUM

You're activating the muscles, reminding them they exist and helping them rebuild.

If you're not sure you're doing it right, or if you're experiencing pain, discomfort during sex or a feeling of pressure down below, ask for a referral to a **pelvic health physio**.

CONTRACEPTION: YOUR EGGS ARE WEARING MINI SKIRTS

Now let's talk contraception. And I'm going to be very honest here.

After you've had your baby, imagine all your eggs wearing miniskirts, lined up at the edge of your ovaries, bending over and waiting for sperm. Biologically? Your body is back in business. Pre-pregnancy, every month, your egg is released, she scans the room, looking for sperm, hoping for the match. When she doesn't find any, she gives up, sheds her lining, and your period arrives. Simple.

Here's what people forget: during pregnancy, that whole system has been on **annual leave**. She's been relaxing. Resting. No ovulation, no pressure. But now? She's back. Fresh, rested, fully dressed and ready to catch *anything* that comes near her. Your body becomes **extremely fertile** after birth – and a lot sooner than you think.

So when I see those TikToks of mums crying with positive pregnancy tests three months postpartum going, 'Oh my God! Oh my God! Oh my God!' I have to ask: Sis . . . how did you think the baby got there? Because fertility doesn't politely wait for you to be ready. It's there. Loud and active. And if you're having sex, even once, you can get pregnant.

This is how we get **Irish twins** – siblings born less than 12 months apart. I'm not saying it's wrong or bad; some people want that, and that's completely fine. But if you *don't*, then we need to talk **contraception** – seriously and without judgement.

During COVID, we actually started offering contraception right there on the postnatal ward because, let's be real, no one had anything else to do. People were going home and getting pregnant again *immediately*. Mummies weren't resting, their bodies weren't recovering, and it was all because no one had a proper conversation about fertility *before* discharge.

Some rely on the **LAM**, the Lactational Amenorrhoea Method. People call it 'breastfeeding as birth control', and while it *can* reduce the chances of pregnancy, it is **not strong enough**. Especially not in those early postnatal months when your body is already extra fertile and your baby's feeding pattern hasn't even stabilised yet. You have to meet *very strict criteria* for LAM to be effective: exclusive breastfeeding, baby under six months, no periods, regular feeding day and night. Miss one feed or introduce a bottle, and the whole thing becomes unreliable. It's a risky game.

So please, talk to your midwife or GP. Ask questions. Think ahead. You don't need to decide right away, but you *do* need to understand your options. Whether it's the pill, the injection, the coil, the implant or condoms, there is something that can work for your lifestyle and your recovery.

POSTPARTUM

UNIQUE EXPERIENCES: TRAUMATIC BIRTH RECOVERY

What if the birth you had wasn't the one you imagined? What if it wasn't what you hoped for, anticipated, dreamt about or even wrote down in your birth plan with so much intention? What if it was traumatic?

I know people mean well when they say things like, *'At least the baby's here and healthy,'* or *'You made it out alive; that's all that matters.'* But let me say this plainly: **your physical health – and your baby's – is the bare minimum**. That should never be the only goal. What we should be hoping for, what we should be planning for, is that you leave that birth not just physically intact, but *mentally okay too*. Because this isn't just about survival, it's about your well-being, your recovery, your future pregnancies, your mental health and your ability to reflect on your birth without flinching.

One thing I always want mums to know is that **you are allowed to talk about your birth**, even if everyone else wants to gloss over it. In fact, it's important that you do. Sometimes, things move so quickly, especially in emergencies, that your *understanding* of what happened never catches up to your *experience* of it. You're just rushed from moment to moment, and then suddenly you're holding a baby with no real idea how you got there. So what can you do?

Before you even leave the hospital, if you're able to, try and have a **debrief**. Ask to speak to the midwife who was present, or the doctor who made certain decisions. Ask them to walk you through what happened. What led to the induction? Why was that intervention necessary? What were the risks? What options were considered? Even if you don't feel ready to process it all, getting the facts now while they're still fresh can be incredibly grounding later. Ask for a copy of your notes if you want. Ask questions, even if your voice shakes.

If your hospital has a **trauma midwife** or a **birth reflections clinic**, you can reach out to them too. These are specific services designed to help you unpack your birth story with someone who understands how physically and emotionally complex it can be. You don't have to be 'in crisis' to access that support; you just need to feel that something about your birth is sitting heavily on you. And if it is? Please don't carry it alone.

If you feel what happened to you was unsafe, disrespectful or unacceptable, and you want to **make a complaint**, that's valid too. It's not dramatic. It's not 'making a fuss'. It's holding systems accountable, and giving your story the weight it deserves. No one has the right to tell you how you *should* feel about what happened to your body.

Because the reality is that when birth trauma goes unspoken, it doesn't just disappear. It often shows up in the next pregnancy, in the fear, in the anxiety, in the mistrust of healthcare professionals, in the dread that history will repeat itself. I don't want that for you.

POSTPARTUM

WHEN YOU SHOULD GO BACK IN – SIGNS THAT NEED MEDICAL ATTENTION

After you've had your baby, whether you gave birth in hospital, at a birth centre or at home, you will usually be given information about what to expect in the days that follow. Your midwife will also check in with you during those early weeks. But in between those visits, it can sometimes feel like you are left to figure things out on your own. And with all the focus naturally on your baby, it's easy to overlook your own recovery.

This list is here to remind you that your body matters too. These are signs and symptoms that mean you need medical attention. If you notice any of them, don't ignore it. Trust your instincts. If something feels off, it is always better to get checked.

- **Headaches and Blurry Vision.** If you're getting persistent headaches (especially ones that don't go away with paracetamol), seeing spots or having changes in your vision, that could be a sign of postnatal pre-eclampsia. Yes, it can still happen *after* birth, even up to six weeks later. Especially if it's paired with swelling in your hands/face or high blood pressure. Call your midwife or GP *immediately*.

- **Heavy Bleeding or Large Clots.** A bit of bleeding is expected (hello, lochia), but **if you're soaking through pads in under an hour,** passing **golf ball-sized clots** or the blood has a **foul smell**, you need to be seen. That could be a sign of retained placenta or infection.
- **High Fever or Flu-Like Symptoms.** A **temperature above 38°C,** feeling feverish or chills, body aches or general 'something's not right' flu symptoms could be a sign of an **infection**, especially in the womb or breasts (mastitis). Call your GP, midwife or go into A&E if needed.
- **Painful, Red, Swollen Breasts.** If one breast is **hot, swollen, sore** and you feel generally unwell, this could be **mastitis**. Continue breastfeeding or expressing if you can, but get medical advice fast. Antibiotics may be needed.
- **Caesarean Scar Issues.** If your **scar becomes red, swollen, starts oozing** or smells bad – that could be an **infection**. Some discomfort is normal, but anything sharp, spreading or increasing after a few days needs checking.
- **Pain or Burning When You Pee.** If peeing stings, burns or you're peeing more often than usual *and* it hurts – that might be a **UTI**. These are common after birth but can spread fast. Always better to treat it early.
- **Shortness of Breath, Chest Pain or Leg Pain.** This one's serious. If you're **short of breath**, have chest

pain or feel pain or swelling in one leg – **go to A&E or call 999**. These could be signs of a **blood clot** (DVT or PE), and they can be life-threatening.
- **Worsening Mood, Anxiety or Disturbing Thoughts.** Your mental health matters too. If you're experiencing **persistent low mood, intrusive thoughts, feeling detached** or having **thoughts of harming yourself or your baby**, it's urgent. Reach out – to your GP, health visitor or emergency services. You are *not* alone.

BREASTFEEDING

If there's one topic I actually hate speaking on, it's breast-feeding. Not because it's not important, but because there are *too many opinions and not nearly enough support* for mums. Everyone has something to say, but when it comes time to actually help you latch a baby onto a sore, engorged boob at 3 a.m., suddenly the room is empty.

Let me be honest with you. Scientifically, breastfeeding is the best option for the baby, for immunity, for bonding. But I will never stand behind guilt-tripping mums, because the truth is that far too many women stop breastfeeding, or never get started, simply because they were not supported. There is this idea that the baby will just come out, latch beautifully, and feed like they read the manual. That is not how it works.

Breastfeeding is a skill for both of you, and learning it takes guidance, patience and real support. If you can, try to get help before you leave the hospital. Ask for time with a midwife or infant feeding specialist, and don't leave until you feel confident. If you have the funds or access, consider seeing a lactation consultant (IBCLC) early on, because it is frustrating to know how amazing breastfeeding can be and then see so many women miss out on it simply because no one gave them the help they needed.

Here's the truth: breastfeeding is a very practical task that needs very practical support. I can give you some general advice, but nothing compares to having someone physically show you what to do. A lot of the challenges at the start are things like sore nipples, engorgement, feeling like you don't have enough milk or worrying that your baby is not latching properly. Positioning is key: chest close to chest, chin tucked into the breast, and the baby's head, neck and body in a straight line. Those are the basics. But again, they are basics you need to see, not just read about.

What I will say is: don't try to figure it all out on your own. There are lactation specialists and midwives who share brilliant content online now. Watching their videos can really help you visualise what a good latch actually looks like. And if you can, speak to a lactation consultant or a trained midwife in person – that is the support that makes the biggest difference.

So yes, I can tell you chest to chest, chin to breast, ear, shoulders and hips in line, but what will help you most is

POSTPARTUM

someone guiding you through it when you are holding your baby. Seek out that practical support early, because it will save you a lot of tears and frustration later.

I always say that breastfeeding is the worst thing to do if it is stealing from you. If every feed leaves you feeling devastated, drained or like you are disappearing into yourself, then it is not worth it. Your mental health matters. Your experience matters. Your bond with your baby is not built solely on milk. Fed is best, and more importantly, supported is better.

While I can say that this is not really my expertise, one person I do want to highlight is an amazing midwife called Olivia Hinge.[24] She is phenomenal at teaching women and families about feeding – any type of feeding – and she shares brilliant content on breastfeeding. If you are looking for clear, practical guidance, I cannot recommend her enough.

IDENTITY SHIFT

Let's talk about the identity shift because it can hit you harder than expected. In Nigeria, especially in the Yoruba tribe, it's common that when a woman gives birth, her name literally changes. She becomes *Iya* (meaning *mother*) [insert child's name] – so if her firstborn is called Tobi, she'd now be called *Iya Tobi*. That name becomes her new identity. If she has twins, she becomes *Iya Ibeji, mother of twins*. Although that might sound like just a sweet tradition, it's deeper than that. It reflects exactly what happens after you give birth. You become known, seen, and often only referred to as someone's mum. Sometimes, in all of that, you start to forget who you were before. Your old name, your old hobbies, your old rhythms - they don't vanish, but they do get buried. Motherhood transforms you, but it can also blur your edges.

It might sound cheesy, but let me tell you the truth: if you're not *intentional* about holding onto the things you love and about reclaiming your identity outside of being a mum, you *will* lose yourself. It's not a maybe. It's not something you can just hope won't happen. Because motherhood has a way of swallowing you whole out of constant need. So if you're not creating space for yourself, the space just won't exist.

I always say this when it comes to relationships, too. People love to say, 'Oh, after a while, the spark fades,' or 'It's normal to just grow apart.' And maybe that's true if you leave it to chance. But me? I'm super intentional in my relationship. I don't *hope* it works - I put in the work. I water the thing I want to grow, and it's exactly the same with motherhood. You can't just hope that you'll still feel like *you* six months in. You have to *fight* for it.

So what do you love? Is it going to the theatre? Cool, maybe you can't go every three months like you used to, but could you go twice a year? Mark it out and protect that time. Do you love painting, reading, dancing, writing, going for a walk in silence? Make a plan. Book the babysitter. Call your mum. Put it in your calendar. If you don't carve out space for

POSTPARTUM

yourself, the world won't hand it to you. Your baby doesn't need a perfect, selfless shell of a mum – they need *you*. Fully. Authentically. Not just someone who meets their needs, but someone who still remembers what lights her up, too.

When a mum does lose her identity in motherhood, people don't always see how deep the ripple effect can go. It's not just about feeling lost in the early days – it can shape how you move through motherhood long-term. When you feel like motherhood robbed you of something – be it your freedom, your dreams, your marriage or your time – it's very easy, without even meaning to, to start placing that weight on your child. Like now they owe you something, or they have to become the success that makes all your sacrifices worth it. That's not fair on them, and it's not fair on you either.

That's why it's so important to catch this early. Be intentional *now*, not later. Because the truth is, yes, you want to be a fantastic mum, but there's no medal coming to say you were the best mum in the whole world. And you losing yourself in the process? That doesn't make you a superhero. You don't get extra points for abandoning everything you loved. You don't need to become a cautionary tale that ends in, 'I gave up everything for you.' You really don't want to become the mum who spends years reminding her child, 'This is what I did for you, this is what I gave up, this is what I had to do.'

Whatever you don't *have* to do? Don't do it. There's no honour in unnecessary struggle. Choose ease where you can. Choose joy where you can. Remember: the best gift you can give your child is a version of you that still remembers who she is.

BOUNCING BACK

You're damned if you do, damned if you don't – that's what it can feel like when it comes to postnatal identity and your body. There's this strange pressure to *miss* your old self, to rush back to who you were before the baby, especially physically. The 'snapback' culture is real. People love to ask, 'When are you going to get your body back?' as if your body has wandered off somewhere and needs retrieving. At the same time, if you *do* decide you want to work on yourself, get back to the gym, eat differently or even post your progress, suddenly there's judgement too. Now you're seen as showing off. Now it's, 'Oh, she's making everyone else feel bad.'

A woman can post online about her abs, share her workout routine and be proud of her progress, and we can still honour *your* journey if your belly hasn't gone anywhere and you haven't even opened the fitness app. It's okay to celebrate someone else without making it a personal attack. It's also okay to take your time, to rest, to heal, and to not care about what your jeans say right now. The world constantly pitches women against each other where there was never really an issue to begin with.

So whether you're the mum who's already lacing up her trainers six weeks postpartum, or the one who's still in mesh underwear, do your thing. Missing your old self is normal. Longing for freedom, for peace, for silence, for a body you recognise – it's all valid. But don't let anyone make you feel like you've failed because your version of 'getting back to you' doesn't look like someone else's.

THE 6-WEEK CHECK-IN

This is supposed to be your *postnatal MOT*. The one that, in theory, gives you space to talk about your physical recovery, mental well-being, contraception, pelvic floor, bleeding, sleep, feeding and anything else that's been on your mind. But let's be honest – **a lot of women leave their six-week check feeling rushed, unheard or like the focus was more on the baby than on them**. Sometimes it's a quick 'How are you?' as the GP scrolls through your notes. Sometimes it's just 'Are you breastfeeding? Any contraception?' and that's it, with barely a glance at your stitches, your scar, your mental state or how you're really coping.

Here's what your six-week check *should* include:

- A conversation about how you're feeling – physically and emotionally.
- Questions about your bleeding, discharge and any pain.
- A check on any stitches or your C-section scar.
- Discussion about your pelvic floor and whether you're having any leaking or pressure.

I'M PREGNANT ... NOW WHAT?

- Chat about sex – yes, it matters, and no, you shouldn't be brushed off if something feels off.
- Contraception options – because, remember, those eggs are ready and waiting.
- Space to talk about your birth – especially if it didn't go to plan.

If you're not offered or asked these things? **Ask. Advocate. Push.**

FIRST WEEKS WITH BABY

I'm going to be totally honest with you – this is a safe space, right? I don't really know much about babies. I really don't. I've always specialised my care around *mummy*, and I always say midwifery literally means 'with woman'.

In most of my work on the labour ward, I see babies for about an hour and a half, tops. After that, they're off with someone whose whole job is baby, not me. So when it comes to in-depth baby care . . . I'm not your girl. I always get loads of emails and questions from mums saying, 'Oh, my three-month-old is doing this,' or 'not doing that,' and once, someone even asked me about a *five-year-old*. I was like, *I have absolutely no clue*. I'm literally as clueless as you are.

But here's what I *do* know, and honestly, I don't think it needs to be much more complicated than this: healthy babies need to be kept clean and warm, they need to be

POSTPARTUM

fed, and they need to be loved. That's it. Everything else is just extra.

REGISTERING YOUR BABY'S BIRTH

Let's talk about registering your baby's birth. Different areas and different countries have their own rules, so check what applies where you live. In the UK, you usually have 42 days (six weeks) to register a birth, and there's actually a fine if you don't do it on time. While you're looking into that, it's also worth checking what financial help might be available to you. Things like Child Benefit, tax credits or other local support schemes can make a difference, and you don't have to wait until you're in the postnatal blur to find out what you qualify for. Research it now so you're not trying to fill out forms with one hand while holding a newborn in the other.

WHAT TO LOOK OUT FOR

I'm going to stick to the first couple of weeks you have your baby at home and the things that are super important to keep an eye on. One of those things is **jaundice**. Jaundice happens when there's too much bilirubin in your baby's blood, and it makes their skin and the whites of their eyes look yellow. In lighter skin, you might notice it most on the face and chest. In Black and Brown babies, it can be harder to spot on the skin, so check the whites of the eyes, the gums and the inside of the lips. We'll always check for jaundice before you leave the hospital, or before your midwife signs off after a home visit, but it can appear a couple of days later. If your baby is extremely sleepy, floppy, not feeding well, peeing dark or doing pale or chalky poos, please get them checked immediately. A little gentle sunlight can also help the body process bilirubin, so don't be afraid to take your baby out for a short walk, even if they're only a few days old.

One thing to know straight away is that it's completely normal for a newborn to **lose a bit of weight** after they're born – even if you're breastfeeding like a pro. They've just come from a world where food was constant and effortless, so it takes a moment for their body to adjust. We usually expect them to be back to their birth weight by around day 10. If they're not, it doesn't automatically mean something is wrong, but it's a sign for your midwife or health visitor to keep a closer eye and offer extra support.

Then there's the **nappies**. Not every baby follows the textbook, but there are some patterns we look for in the early days. In the first couple of days, poos are dark and sticky – that's meconium, which is baby's first poo, made up of all the things they swallowed in the womb. Over the next few days, as feeding gets established, those poos should start turning lighter, looser and eventually mustard-yellow if you're breastfeeding (formula-fed babies may have poos that are more tan or brown). A good rule of thumb: if baby is feeding well and you're seeing an increasing number of wet

POSTPARTUM

and dirty nappies each day in the first week, that's reassuring. It tells us their digestive system is working.

Another thing that happens in those early days is the **newborn blood spot test**, also known as the heel prick test. This is usually done on day five and screens for a few rare but serious conditions, including sickle cell. In the NHS, the rule is generally: if you don't hear anything back, it means everything came back normal. The test itself is just a tiny prick on your baby's heel, but yes, some babies will cry (and some will barely flinch). If hearing your baby cry makes your heart ache, here's a tip: put them to the breast or give them a bottle during the test. Feeding can be a great distraction and helps calm them, and you might find they don't even notice what's happening.

In that first week, you're still figuring each other out, so keep it simple. For cord care, clean it gently with cooled boiled or distilled water, keep it dry, and fold nappies down so it's not rubbing or getting damp – especially with boys, who can surprise you mid-change. For nappies in general, change them often, let the skin dry before popping a fresh one on, and use a thin layer of barrier cream if you notice any redness starting.

When it comes to clothing, the 'one extra layer than you' rule is a good guide, but check the back of your baby's neck to really know. Warm and dry is perfect – sweaty means they're too hot. If they cry a lot, remember this is their only language right now; sometimes it's hunger, sometimes comfort, sometimes wind. Try skin-to-skin, gentle rocking or a soft shush in their ear.

Tummy time in week one can simply be them lying on your chest while you're relaxing – it's bonding time for you and gentle muscle work for them. Most of all, trust yourself. You'll get to know your baby's cues quicker than you think.

SAFE SLEEPING: COT OR CO-SLEEPING

I'll be honest – this isn't my favourite topic to talk about. It's one of those areas where opinions are split, people get defensive and the conversation can get heated. But where your baby sleeps matters. The research is clear that the safest place for your baby to sleep is in their own cot or Moses basket, on a firm, flat mattress, in the same room as you for at least the first six months. That setup significantly reduces the risk of SIDS (Sudden Infant Death Syndrome). That being said, we know that many parents end up bed-sharing – sometimes by choice, sometimes because it's the only way anyone gets any sleep – and research has shifted from 'never do it' to 'if you do it, here's how to make it safer'. This shift happened because they found that parents were already doing it but not always following safe guidance, so instead of just saying 'don't', the focus is now on harm reduction.

If you do decide to co-sleep, or find yourself doing it, you must follow these safety tips:

- Baby should sleep on their back, on a firm, flat, clutter-free surface.
- No pillows, toys, bumpers or loose blankets near baby.

POSTPARTUM

- Tuck a lightweight blanket around them, no higher than shoulder level, with their hands free.
- Keep the bed clear of other children or pets, and ensure there's no gap where baby could fall or become trapped.
- Never co-sleep on a sofa or armchair.
- Never co-sleep if you or your partner have had alcohol, taken drugs, are extremely tired or if your baby was premature or had a low birth weight.
- If you smoke – even if you don't smoke in the bedroom – you should not be co-sleeping at all, as smoking significantly increases the risk of SIDS.

Ultimately, I believe a baby is safest in their own cot, but if they are in your bed, it's about following the rules that keep them as safe as possible. I've also seen how hard it can be for some mums who've tried and tried to settle their baby in the cot, only to be met with hours of crying and no rest for anyone. It's easy to read the research, but it's another thing to live through night after night of exhaustion. That's why, from the very beginning, I always suggest trying to keep your baby in their cot and seeing how they get on, because if they settle well there from the start, it's often easier to maintain.

BABY'S FIRST BATH

When your baby is first born, you don't need to rush to scrub off all that vernix (the creamy white coating on their skin) – it's great for temperature regulation and skin protection. The NHS also recommends waiting before the first bath, and keeping it gentle when you do.

Make sure the room is warm, the water is around 37 °C, and you have everything you need to hand before you start. You don't have to bathe your baby every day. Topping and tailing with cotton wool and warm water is fine in between.

When you do bathe them, support their head and shoulders at all times. Start with their face and hair, then move on to the rest of the body. Dry them quickly and keep them warm. Some parents find it easier to wash the head first, pop on a hat, and then bathe the body.

Every culture has its own traditions around baby's first bath. Some do it straight away, some wait a week or more. There's no one right way. For clear, evidence-based guidance, I'd always recommend going to the NHS website and searching 'NHS washing and bathing your baby'.[25] It's a solid, trusted resource you can follow step by step.

And that's it, folks – that's me done with what I know about babies. There's a whole world of research and resources out there, and I love that you're reading this book, but you'll probably also want to read a book that's fully about babies too. This is just my lane.

My advice? Don't let anyone overcomplicate things for you. Your baby's core needs are simple: fed, clean and loved. You can do that. Don't get distracted by the 'fold your clothes like this' brigade, or the 'you must use this exact brand' crowd. Remember – a lot of brands thrive off the fact that mums want to be good mums. They push the idea that the more expensive the item, the more you must love your baby. That's nonsense. Work within your capacity. If you check the labels, you'll often find supermarket products have the same ingredients as the pricey, 'premium' stuff. Your worth as a mum isn't measured by receipts.

LOOK AT YOU – YOU DID IT

If you've made it here, first of all, thank you. What a journey. You've carried so much, learned so much, and hopefully laughed a little too. Writing this book has been one of the most special things I've ever done, and knowing that it's been part of *your* journey means more than I can say.

When I started this book, I said I wanted it to feel like a warm hug when nothing else does. I hope, somewhere in these pages, it has done exactly that. I hope it's helped you feel seen, informed, comforted and maybe even entertained on the days where you just needed a bit of realness.

Pregnancy is huge – physically, emotionally, mentally, spiritually. You've been stretched in ways you didn't think possible, and I need you to pause and acknowledge that. The strength it takes to grow, carry and bring life into the world is not small. It's sacred. It's extraordinary. And it's yours.

I hope this book has given you a few 'aha' moments, made you nod along, or even made you feel less alone when things got confusing or heavy. More than anything, I hope it's left you feeling empowered – like you know your body, your choices and your voice matter. Because they do.

Whether this is your first pregnancy or your fifth, whether things went exactly as planned or nothing like you expected, please know this: you did it. You've already done something incredible. Thank you for letting me be part of your story, for trusting me to walk with you through such a transformative time.

You've got this – and I've got you.

ENDNOTES

PART 1
THE FIRST TRIMESTER

1. Lundgren, S. et al. 'Plasma volume expansion across healthy pregnancy: A systematic review and meta-analysis', *BMC Pregnancy and Childbirth*, vol. 19 (2019), p. 464. https://bmcpregnancychildbirth.biomedcentral.com/articles/10.1186/s12884-019-2619-6
2. Abd El-Ghaffar, N. M. et al. 'Prevalence of MTHFR gene mutation in pregnant women and its correlation with pregnancy complications', *Journal of Genetic Disorders and Genetic Reports*, vol. 12 (2023), pp. 1–8. https://journals.lww.com/md-journal/fulltext/2020/11060/prevalence_of_the_methylenetetrahydrofolate.17.aspx
3. Bošković, A. et al. 'Association of MTHFR polymorphism, folic acid, and vitamin B12 with serum homocysteine levels in pregnant women', *Biomolecules and Biomedicine*, vol. 24 (2024), pp. 138–43. https://pmc.ncbi.nlm.nih.gov/articles/PMC10787622/

4. Czeizel, A. E. and Dudas, I. 'Prevention of the first occurrence of neural-tube defects by periconceptional vitamin supplementation', *The New England Journal of Medicine*, vol. 327, no. 26 (1992), pp. 1832-5. www.nejm.org/doi/full/10.1056/NEJM199212243272602

5. Deganich, M. et al. 'Toxoplasmosis infection during pregnancy', *Tropical Medicine and Infectious Disease*, vol. 8, no. 1 (2022), p. 3. https://pmc.ncbi.nlm.nih.gov/articles/PMC9862191/

6. Tam, C. et al. 'Food-borne illnesses during pregnancy: Prevention and treatment', *Canadian Family Physician*, vol. 56, no. 4 (2010), pp. 341-3. www.ncbi.nlm.nih.gov/pmc/articles/PMC2860824/

7. Brazier, Yvette. 'All you need to know about salmonella', *Medical News Today*, 2020, updated 2024. www.medicalnewstoday.com/articles/160942

8. Institute of Food Science and Technology. 'New advice on eating runny eggs – Food Standards Agency', 2017. www.ifst.org/news/new-advice-eating-runny-eggs-fsa-0

9. Centers for Disease Control and Prevention (CDC). 'Clinical overview of listeriosis', 2023. https://www.cdc.gov/listeria/hcp/clinical-overview/index.html

10. Davidson P. W. et al. 'Prenatal methyl mercury exposure from fish consumption and child development: A review of evidence and perspectives from the Seychelles Child Development Study', *Neurotoxicology*, vol 6 (2006) pp. 1106-09. https://pubmed.ncbi.nlm.nih.gov/16687174/

11. 'Advice about eating fish', *U.S. Food and Drug Administration (FDA)*, 2021. www.fda.gov/food/consumers/advice-about-eating-fish

12. Bastos Maia, S. et al. 'Vitamin A and pregnancy: A narrative review', *Nutrients*, vol. 11, no. 3 (2019), p. 681. https://pmc.ncbi.nlm.nih.gov/articles/PMC6470929/

ENDNOTES

13. 'Foods to avoid in pregnancy', *NHS UK*, 2023. www.nhs.uk/pregnancy/keeping-well/foods-to-avoid/
14. Li, J. et al. 'A meta-analysis of risk of pregnancy loss and caffeine and coffee consumption during pregnancy', *Public Health Nutrition*, vol. 18, no. 4 (2015), pp. 692–700. www.sciencedirect.com/science/article/abs/pii/S0020729215002684

PART 3
THE THIRD TRIMESTER

15. Alwan, N. A. et al. 'Why are black women still more likely to die in childbirth?', *British Medical Journal*, vol. 388 (2025), r226. www.bmj.com/content/388/bmj.r226

PART 4
THE BIG PUSH (LITERALLY)

16. Kibuka, M. 'Evaluating the effects of maternal positions in childbirth: An overview of Cochrane systematic reviews', *European Journal of Midwifery*, vol. 5, no. 57 (2021). www.europeanjournalofmidwifery.eu/Evaluating-the-effects-of-maternal-positions-in-childbirth-An-overview-of-Cochrane,142781,0,2.html
17. Lawrence, A., Lewis, L., Hofmeyr, G. J. et al. 'Maternal positions and mobility during first stage labour', *Cochrane Database of Systematic Reviews*, vol. 8 (2013), CD003934. www.cochranelibrary.com/cdsr/doi/10.1002/14651858.CD003934.pub3/full
18. Hunter S., Hofmeyr G. J. and Kulier R. 'Hands and knees posture in late pregnancy or labour for fetal malposition (lateral or posterior)', *Cochrane Database of Systematic Reviews*, vol. 4, (2007), CD001063. www.cochranelibrary.com/cdsr/doi/10.1002/14651858.CD001063.pub3/full

19. Jayawardana, S. et al. 'Association of squatting activities of pregnant women during the later stages with labour outcomes: A descriptive study', *Journal of Anthropology and Archaeology*, vol. 11 (2023), pp. 1-11. www.scirp.org/journal/paperinformation?paperid=131437.
20. Aslantaş, B. N. and Çankaya, S. 'The effect of birth ball exercise on labor pain, delivery duration, birth comfort and birth satisfaction: A randomized controlled study', *Archives of Gynecology and Obstetrics*, vol. 309, no. 6 (2024), pp. 2459-74. https://doi.org/10.1007/s00404-023-07115-4
21. Kibuka, M. 'Evaluating the effects of maternal positions in childbirth: An overview of Cochrane systematic reviews', *European Journal of Midwifery*, vol. 5, no. 57 (2021). www.europeanjournalofmidwifery.eu/Evaluating-the-effects-of-maternal-positions-in-childbirth-An-overview-of-Cochrane,142781,0,2.html
22. Cronin, R. S., Li, M., Thompson, J. M. D. et al. 'An individual participant data meta-analysis of maternal going-to-sleep position, interactions with fetal vulnerability, and the risk of late stillbirth', *EClinicalMedicine*, vol. 10 (2019), pp. 49-57. www.thelancet.com/journals/eclinm/article/PIIS2589-5370(19)30054-9/fulltext.
23. Maternal Mental Health Alliance. www.maternalmentalhealthalliance.org

PART 5
POSTPARTUM

24. www.oliviahinge.com
25. 'Washing and bathing your baby', *NHS UK*, 2024. www.nhs.uk/baby/caring-for-a-newborn/washing-and-bathing-your-baby/

GLOSSARY

Anti-D

Anti-D is an injection given to people who are rhesus (RhD) negative during pregnancy or after birth to prevent their immune system from developing antibodies against rhesus-positive blood.

Breech

When the baby's bottom or feet are facing down instead of the head. Sometimes babies turn before labour starts, but if not, your healthcare team will discuss safe birth options with you.

Cord clamping

When the umbilical cord is clamped and cut after birth. Some parents choose to delay clamping for a short while so that more blood flows from the placenta to the baby.

CTG (Cardiotocography)
A test used during pregnancy and labour to monitor your baby's heartbeat and your contractions. The goal is to check how your baby is coping — for example, whether their heart rate changes in response to contractions or movements. It's usually done using two round sensors strapped to your bump.

Down syndrome (Trisomy 21)
A genetic condition caused by an extra copy of chromosome 21. It's associated with some level of learning disability and certain physical features, but many people with Down syndrome live long, fulfilling lives.

Edwards' syndrome (Trisomy 18)
A rare but serious genetic condition caused by an extra copy of chromosome 18. It can lead to severe developmental delays and health complications.

Episiotomy
A small cut made in the perineum (the area between the vagina and anus) to help deliver the baby if the tissue isn't stretching easily or if the baby needs to come out quickly.

Forceps
Smooth, curved metal instruments that look like large tongs. They're used to gently help deliver the baby's head if pushing alone isn't enough.

GLOSSARY

Gestational diabetes

A type of diabetes that develops during pregnancy and usually goes away after birth. It means your body struggles to manage blood sugar levels effectively while pregnant.

Induction of labour

When labour is started artificially rather than waiting for it to begin on its own. This can be done using a pessary, gel or a hormone drip to encourage contractions.

Membrane sweep

A technique where a midwife or doctor gently sweeps a finger around the cervix to help release hormones (prostaglandins) that may trigger labour.

Neural tube defects

A group of conditions that occur when the neural tube (the structure that develops into the brain and spinal cord) does not close properly in early pregnancy, usually within the first four weeks.

Patau's syndrome (Trisomy 13)

A rare genetic condition caused by an extra copy of chromosome 13. It can cause serious physical and developmental problems.

Perineum

The area of skin and muscle between the vagina and the anus. It naturally stretches during birth, and sometimes may tear or need stitches afterwards.

Placenta
An organ that grows in the womb during pregnancy. It connects to your baby via the umbilical cord, providing oxygen and nutrients while removing waste.

Placenta praevia
Where the placenta is positioned low in the uterus and partially or completely covers the cervix (the opening to the womb).

Pre-eclampsia
A condition that can develop in pregnancy, usually after 20 weeks. It causes high blood pressure and can affect the kidneys, liver and placenta. It's monitored closely because it can be serious if left untreated.

Rhesus status (Rh status)
Refers to whether your blood has a specific protein (called the Rhesus D antigen) on the surface of your red blood cells. If you have it, you're Rhesus positive (Rh+); if not, you're Rhesus negative (Rh-). This becomes important in pregnancy because it can affect how your body reacts to your baby's blood type.

Ventouse
A suction cup attached to the baby's head to help guide them out during birth, usually when a little extra assistance is needed in the final stage of labour.

RESOURCES

NHS UK, 'Pregnancy', https://www.nhs.uk/pregnancy/

NHS UK, 'Foods to avoid in pregnancy', https://www.nhs.uk/pregnancy/keeping-well/foods-to-avoid/

Selondonics, 'Tasty recipes when you have gestational diabetes', https://www.selondonics.org/wp-content/uploads/gestational-diabetes-recipe-book.pdf

Tommy's, 'Is it serious? Pregnancy symptom checker', https://www.tommys.org/pregnancy-information/symptom-checker

Olivia Hinge, *A Judgement-Free Guide to Feeding Your Baby: Boob, Bottle and All*, (Yellow Kite, 2024)

Emily Oster, *Expecting Better*, (Penguin Press, 2013)

ACKNOWLEDGEMENTS

First and always, I want to thank God. At sixteen, I had a vivid dream of myself delivering a baby. I woke up confused, laughing at the idea that I would ever be a midwife. And yet here I am, years later, not only having lived that dream but writing a whole book about it. God planted the seed long before I understood it, and He guided every step that brought me here. In all things, I thank Him.

To my man, my man, my man, you carried me through this entire process. Truly. The sleepless nights, the mood swings, the deadlines, the self doubt, the moments where I asked you if any of this made sense. You believed in me when I was tired, reminded me I was capable when I felt overwhelmed, and loved me with a patience I will never take for granted. Thank you for being my grounding, my comfort and my constant reminder that I can do this.

To my family, thank you for being the backbone I did not even know I needed while writing this. The encouragement, the prayers, the check-ins, the love, I felt all of it. And to Anna and Esther, my girls, thank you for the endless video calls, listening to chapter after chapter, giving me energy when I had none left and hyping me when I needed it the most.

To my agents, Zoe and Olivia, thank you. Zoe, thank you for seeing my videos and thinking I might actually have a book in me. I am so glad you reached out to me, because that message changed everything. And Olivia, thank you for supporting me through this entire process with so much care and confidence. I am deeply grateful for both of you.

To my management team, Charlotte, Rianna, Chims and Fran, thank you for stepping in exactly when I needed you. You all carried everything outside of these pages so I could focus on the pages. Thank you for organising me, encouraging me and handling the madness with so much grace.

To Kat, my midwifery manager, thank you for believing in me from day one. You taught me how to be a midwife. You taught me how to deliver babies. You taught me how to stand in a room and trust my own skills. You shaped so much of the midwife I became inside the NHS and I will always be grateful for your leadership, your guidance and the faith you had in me. Thank you for showing me that I could be a midwife inside the NHS and still be a midwife outside it.

To the NHS, you made me strong. You shaped the midwife I became, taught me resilience, stretched me, challenged me and gifted me with experiences that live in every chapter of this book.

ACKNOWLEDGEMENTS

To the HarperCollins team, thank you for taking a chance on me. And Julia, thank you for every email, every bit of guidance and every moment of support. Thank you for letting me add things, adjust things and sneak in extra lines after my deadline. You have been patient, kind and such a joy to work with.

To the mother community, every woman who has trusted me with her pregnancy, her birth, her fears, her joy and her questions, thank you. You inspire me every single day. You are the reason I teach, the reason I speak and the reason I continue to show up.

To my social media community, every single person who follows, supports, shares, comments and sends love, thank you for creating a space where women feel safe, educated and empowered. Your support has carried me more than you will ever know.

And finally, thank you to you, the person holding this book. Thank you for opening these pages, for trusting my words and for letting me be part of your journey.

ABOUT THE AUTHOR

Elizabeth Idowu, professionally known as Mamadinya, is a qualified midwife, educator and advocate dedicated to making pregnancy education clear, relatable and empowering. She began her career in nursing but returned to midwifery after realising it was the calling she had felt since sixteen, when she dreamed of delivering a baby.

Working in the labour ward, Elizabeth quickly saw how many women were entering birth without the knowledge they needed to make informed choices. Determined to bridge that gap, she began creating content that blended medical insight with humour, clarity and compassion. Her work has since reached more than 600,000 people across her platforms.

Elizabeth is the founder of Mama's Classes, an educational platform teaching women the realities of labour and birth. She also created Bumps and Brunches, a global pregnancy-only event series built to provide expectant mothers with community, support and evidence-based information in a space designed entirely for them.

Her commitment to improving maternity experiences led her to launch Mama's Perinatal Allies, a training programme that equips people to support women through pregnancy, birth and the postnatal period. Elizabeth is especially passionate about advocating for Black women and ensuring they receive the safe, respectful care they deserve.

Elizabeth continues to teach, create and support women through her work, always centred on education, empowerment and community.